WALKING TOGETHER, WALKING FAR

WALKING TOGETHER, WALKING FAR

HOW A U.S. AND AFRICAN MEDICAL SCHOOL PARTNERSHIP IS WINNING THE FIGHT AGAINST HIV/AIDS

FRAN QUIGLEY

WITH A FOREWORD BY PAUL FARMER

INDIANA UNIVERSITY PRESS
BLOOMINGTON AND INDIANAPOLIS

This book is a publication of

Indiana University Press
601 North Morton Street
Bloomington, IN 47404-3797 USA

http://iupress.indiana.edu

Telephone orders   800-842-6796
Fax orders   812-855-7931
Orders by e-mail   iuporder@indiana.edu

⊚The paper used in this publication meets the minimum
requirements of the American National Standard
for Information Sciences—Permanence of Paper for
Printed Library Materials, ANSI Z39.48-1992.

Manufactured in the United States of America

Library of Congress Cataloging-in-Publication Data

Quigley, Fran, date
  Walking together, walking far : how a U.S. and African medical
school partnership is winning the fight against HIV/AIDS /
Fran Quigley ; foreword by Paul Farmer.
      p. cm.
  Includes index.
  ISBN 978-0-253-35324-5 (cloth : alk. paper) —
  ISBN 978-0-253-22089-9 (pbk. : alk. paper)
  1. Indiana University School of Medicine. 2. Moi University.
School of Medicine. 3. AIDS (Disease)—Kenya. 4. AIDS
(Disease)—Treatment—International cooperation. I. Title.
  RA643.86.K4Q85 2009
  362.196'9792—dc22
                                           2008043193

1 2 3 4 5 14 13 12 11 10 09

IF YOU WANT TO WALK FAST,
WALK ALONE. IF YOU WANT TO
WALK FAR, WALK TOGETHER.

AFRICAN PROVERB

CONTENTS

FOREWORD

WALKING TOGETHER, WALKING FAR IS surely the best title that could be devised for a book about people from two very different nations, coming together to fight AIDS. Fran Quigley has done a superb job in describing what is, on the face of it, a straightforward collaboration between an American academic medical center and another one in Africa. Hundreds of similar collaborations link academic institutions on the two continents, in addition to thousands, if not tens of thousands, of bicontinental AIDS programs of other kinds. With so much experience on tap, it is unfortunate that so many lessons remain to be learned about the process of "accompaniment," as walking together is termed in theological circles. For if projects that link the rich world—any American university would qualify as such—to the poorer reaches of the developing world are to succeed, then learning to walk together must become a key goal of such connections. But this book is about much more than teamwork in the face of a devastating illness that happens to be the leading killer of young adults in Western Kenya. More importantly, it's about the epiphanies experienced by some of the heroes in the book, and about how they acted, and continue to act, on these epiphanies. It's about how these protagonists decided to walk together with Kenyan colleagues, students, patients, and sundry family members.

This, then, is a book about awakenings and transformations as much as it is about a partnership between a U.S. and an African medical school, with implications for just about anyone seeking to understand the ways in which global structural inequalities, the chief reason that AIDS is prevalent in some areas and rare in others, undermine good-will efforts to take on disease and poverty. There is no shortage of these efforts, but rather a growing enthusiasm for them, especially among students. One recent piece in the Washington *Post* observes that "For a Global Generation, Public Health Is a Hot Field," and this is a book that should be read by every student of public health.

It would be easy to make these claims in a sweeping fashion, but I'd like to explore them in the down-to-earth style in which this book is written. "Accompaniment" is precisely the notion that has driven forward our own work in Haiti, Peru, Rwanda, Malawi, Lesotho, Burundi, Boston, and elsewhere. "Walking together" is as good a term as any—as long as all parties concerned can walk. Not everyone in this book can walk; not everyone walks out alive. But the reason this book is such an important contribution is that it is about a group of people who questioned received wisdom about what is possible in treating the destitute sick.

It's also a book about the power, and limitations, of empathy. Imagine that you are a doctor or a nurse. Imagine that you are from Indiana, but understand that the place you call home is only one of many salient facts about you. Others include the ability to see humanity in every face, and especially in the face of those sick with treatable afflictions but too poor to obtain them. In many ways, this book tells the story of Dr. Joe Mamlin, a professor of medicine at Indiana University. Mamlin was, we read, "seeking to put the finishing touches" on his career, a successful one by any standard. He'd had previous experience in Kenya, and was planning to spend a couple of years as a clinician-teacher at the Moi University School of Medicine, which had long had a formal relationship with his home university in the United States. But his work in Western Kenya, one of the epicenters of the AIDS pandemic, made it increasingly difficult for him to say goodbye to medicine or to Kenya. The wards of the nascent teaching hospital were full of dying young people, including a student named Daniel Ochieng.

At the outset, in the fall of 2000, Ochieng was one of millions of nameless and faceless people suffering in obscurity, dying from AIDS. How, then, do we even know his name and see his photograph in this wonderful book? As a physician working in the poorest reaches of the world, I can recognize the scene Quigley so vividly describes: one of Mamlin's fifth-year students, Bernard Olayo, was in the hospital ward later in the day than usual (the exact time is worth noting since many young doctors, bereft of the medicines needed to treat these patients, would flee those wards at the earliest possible moment). Mamlin saw Olayo and asked: Why are you still here? Mamlin was shocked to learn that the skeletal figure by whom Olayo was sitting was another medical student—one of their own. An epiphany, beautifully described by Quigley, ensued: if we can't even help our own students, Mamlin concluded, maybe we should pack it up and go home.

Mamlin and his colleagues stayed in Eldoret and together with their Kenyan colleagues built one of Africa's largest and most important AIDS-treatment programs. We owe a great deal to Ochieng, since he humanized the face of AIDS for some on the Indiana team. The thousands of Kenyans dying of AIDS at that moment now had a name: Daniel. If Daniel died, a potential physician died, leaving Kenya in more desperate shape than before. This epiphany and recognition led Mamlin and others to question the then-regnant orthodoxy—that it was not "cost-effective" to treat AIDS in Africa—and to push forward the treatment and training and outreach programs described in this book. AMPATH ended up benefiting not only the Daniels—members of our own tribe of students, doctors, and professionals—but thousands of the truly nameless poor who faced much worse fates (and deeper invisibility) since they suffered from the same disease but were unlikely to have medical students paying special attention to their suffering. Thus did the travails of a young man who, in spite of his humble background, would be regarded as a member of the elite by the local poor lead not only to an awakening of empathy among the Americans who are the protagonists of this book, but also to the strengthening of empathy among young Kenyan students.

In Quigley's account, we catch more than a glimpse of the objections raised to treating Daniel. It's a long list; it caused a great deal of delay. We in the field know such arguments well because they were often used as blunt instruments to discourage discussion of programs such as AMPATH: it is irrational and wasteful, it was long argued, to treat AIDS in resource-poor settings. We lack the infrastructure, other experts objected. It's not sustainable, said some; treating AIDS will draw resources away from other priorities in public health. There were even those who argued that it was not "culturally appropriate" to treat AIDS, as

Africans were alleged to have "a different concept of time." An entire book could be devoted to the long list of reasons for inaction. Whatever the reason, inaction led to only one outcome, for there was only one thing that could have saved the young student's life, and that was access to the same standard of care for AIDS that prevails in Indiana: antiretroviral drugs.

This may seem an obvious point to some readers. After all, there is no other treatment for AIDS, and the wards of Eldoret were full of people languishing with this same diagnosis. Why and how might this obvious conclusion be termed an epiphany? In this regard, Quigley's is a frank book. Honest accounts of programs such as AMPATH—projects that exist all over the world—are too rarely encountered. Prior to the disbursement of its first pill, praise for the collaboration, as Quigley notes, flowed from every imaginable source. Quigley even suggests that the praise allowed some, including Mamlin and many others whom we meet in these pages, to expect real results. The awkward fact about this international medical initiative was that until Daniel Ochieng came along this much-praised collaboration, like almost all comparable programs at that time, was not treating the number one cause of death in the area in which it functioned. As is noted honestly in this book, Ochieng himself knew nothing about the treatment for his disease because it had been concluded, by "the experts," that this treatment could not be provided to Africans. As Quigley notes, not a single patient at the Moi Teaching and Referral Hospital had ever received antiretroviral treatment—many years after it was the standard of care in the affluent world. Daniel Ochieng, alive and well today because he was recognized as a colleague and a peer, is certain that he was the only person with HIV/AIDS to walk out of his ward alive in 2000.

In truth, anyone who moves between the resource-rich world of an American university and a city in Africa quickly sees not only the lack of resources necessary to practice modern medicine, but also, and more perniciously, a double standard for treatment of AIDS, malignancies, epilepsy, mental illness, and a host of other complex illnesses that afflict the poor just as much, or more, than they afflict those who do not live in poverty. This is why it is possible to observe, as Mamlin does in this book, that "it is easy to sit in a conference room and say it is not wise to provide treatment here." Think about this sentence and ask the unposed question: why on earth would it be easy to sit in a conference room, anywhere in the world, and argue that it is "not wise" to provide treatment for the leading killer of young people?

If empathy served to reveal the untenable nature of such double standards, it is important to note that the work described in this book is not built only upon the foundations of empathy. It is built upon many other strengths. Among these are solidarity (perhaps the noblest of human sentiments); commitment; pity and mercy (sentiments not to be scorned in this age); curiosity about problems new and old; the desire to be effective as a clinician and teacher (or student); and even love (of learning, of others, of using the tools that science gives us). The work of AMPATH is also founded on a new and better way of understanding how clinical medicine and public health can work together to confront novel challenges. Asking the unasked question led AMPATH to walk together with the Daniel Ochiengs of the world but also, as the rest of the book's title would suggest, to walk far.

For one thing, the birth of AMPATH forced this book's protagonists to think hard about how best to approach broader development efforts, which are examined in Chapter 6. Few doctors have ever grappled with these sorts of problems; we were not trained to do so. When Joe Mamlin discovered that one in five of his patients were having difficulty finding food, he was probably under-diagnosing the problem, if experience in more rural reaches of Western Kenya is relevant to Eldoret. But discovering the problem led the AMPATH team to act: just as antiretrovirals are the only treatment for AIDS, food is the only known treatment for malnutrition. Feeding 30,000 a week is surely one of the victories of which Mamlin and AMPATH should be most proud, since this sort of effort, unstintingly praised by the hungry, is also dismissed by development experts and even some public-health specialists. In Rwanda, a colleague denounced our own efforts to make sure that those with wasting consumptive diseases, and hospitalized patients, had access to food: this was critiqued as "promoting dependency." But all humans are dependent on food, and great food insecurity is, like an epidemic, an emergency that requires prompt action, not hairsplitting over potential "moral hazard."

AMPATH has taken the socioeconomic challenges of Africa seriously, and one of the best parts of this book is its exploration of local efforts to integrate patients—once bed-ridden ("down" as they say in Kenya) and now well—into income-generating activities. Surely this is not something that Mamlin or the other physicians, Kenyan or American, were trained to do any more than I was, but once the fateful decision to treat AIDS was taken, a longer walk was bound to follow.

It's no small feat to walk away from the defeatist views of a decade ago and toward the optimism of Joe Mamlin and his colleagues, but their change of direction is now more and more common across Africa. *Walking Together, Walking Far* lays out the broader international context that conditioned the growth of AMPATH. After years of hand-wringing and nay-saying, during which the self-described expert consensus was that AIDS treatment was not feasible in poor countries, the Global Fund to Fight AIDS, Tuberculosis, and Malaria was born; shortly thereafter, the President's Emergency Plan for AIDS Relief (PEPFAR) came along, and a vigorous effort to see three million people in developing countries on treatment by 2005 was being coordinated at the World Health Organization. Historians may quibble as to their exact order and causality, but the main factors were these.

Anyone who tells you that PEPFAR and similar programs have only created problems is surely not a patient or a clinician. Of course there are problems and challenges, and many of them are evident in this book. I'd like to underline four that strike me as worthy of special attention. This is a book about walking together, but we have yet to walk far enough: we have a long, long way to go before we achieve any sort of equipoise between rich-world academic institutions and those whose missions include service to the destitute sick in Africa or elsewhere. Put another way, does it make sense for such disparate settings as a city in Indiana and a city in Western Kenya to be linked in a strictly "academic" relationship? The answer to that question, as laid out here, is no. For the chief duties of academic medicine cannot fail to include service to the poor—the very people who die, whether in a hospital in Eldoret or, more likely, in their own dirt-floored homes. If we fail to provide the best available service to those people, then we will all be reduced, in the words of one young Kenyan physician, to mortuary attendants. What gave birth to this project, and this book, was the realization that double standards of care—one for the poor and one for the rich, or one for Americans and another for Africans—were not tenable in a transnational project. Nor are they tenable anywhere, not as standards or policy goals, on our increasingly interconnected planet.

As AMPATH grows rapidly, it faces what are termed, in public health, programmatic challenges. In 2001, shortly after Daniel Ochieng became the first patient to receive proper treatment in the program, it was possible to follow all patients and to lose none of them "to follow-up," in medical jargon. Now, as AMPATH balloons in response to vast and previously unacknowledged need, up to a quarter of newly enrolled patients may be lost to follow-up. In my view, there is only one way to proceed, and that is to support community-based accompaniment that is done not only through mobile clinics but by training and salarying community health workers. My own trips to another part of Western Kenya introduced me to the widespread social fiction of "community health volunteers"—people who are charged with accompanying patients but who are not given the support necessary to do so. Poor themselves, they can ill afford to volunteer, and so loss-to-follow-up is high throughout PEPFAR-funded programs that do not stipend community health workers, even modestly.

Another programmatic challenge is integrating what are termed "vertical" programs to diagnose and treat AIDS, tuberculosis, and malaria with broader efforts to strengthen health systems. Instead of continuing a false debate about whether or not programs like AMPATH weaken health systems by sucking up resources and personnel, we should ask how we can use these more vertical efforts to draw long-overdue attention and resources to the host of health problems faced in places like Eldoret and surrounding towns and villages.

Third, "brain drain" is a far more complex topic than is usually acknowledged. We hear about one talented American doctor who vowed never to return to Africa because of what he could not achieve without the tools of the trade: the right diagnostics, preventives, and therapeutics. We also read that one hospital ward was called "Bosnia" because its situation was regarded as so hopeless. Why the despair? Because so many of these patients, most of them young, had two treatable diseases: tuberculosis and AIDS. Daniel Ochieng, like so many others, was also afflicted by tuberculosis. His classmates were reduced to tears when tuberculosis and AIDS reduced him to 72 pounds. The reader lauds their empathy and is grateful for it. But it is important to acknowledge that Daniel almost underwent precisely the fate reserved for the majority of their patients: AIDS, tuberculosis, wasting, and death. And what clinician would want to work in a setting in which the tools to respond are well known but unavailable? Helping Kenyan professionals confront their own responsibilities to the poor of their country is important, but as AMPATH shows, they must be furnished with the tools of their trade.

Many other important issues remain—for example, the proper protocols for the prevention of mother-to-child transmission of HIV and an honest assessment of failures of implementation—but these can be taken up in professional journals and in conference rooms. How the rich world interacts with the poor world is the most important question that comes out of reading Quigley's wonderful and affecting account. Understandably, not everyone will like the stark terms in which this question is posed here. Quigley's discussion introduces many of the inescapable complexities. We meet doctors who are aware of the debates—"do we teach a man to fish or do we give him fish?"—but who know too little of the unfairness of international trade regimes. We meet people who complain about the cost of drugs but who are in the dark about how the pharmaceutical industry works. We meet physicians who focus on AIDS but not tuberculosis, even though these two diseases are inseparable in Kenya (as in the rest of the world). We meet people who understand that the root causes of these epidemics are social—poverty, migration, et cetera—but who are ill-equipped to respond to such large-scale problems. As one person notes, "it all takes money to fix these things." Indeed: it takes money to lessen poverty; food to lessen hunger;

medicines to lessen deaths from AIDS; operating suites to address obstructed labor, and so on. But it also takes passion and, above all, vision, and that is what the leaders of this program allowed to flourish and encouraged in others.

So to return to the question, posed so eloquently by Quigley, Can foreign aid work? Of course it can. But it can work only when linked to sound analyses of local need; to a broader vision in which "aid" would be replaced by solidarity; and to robust skepticism about facile notions of sustainability, cost-effectiveness, and feasibility. *Walking Together, Walking Far* describes one such effort in detail and with candor. For both the example and the account, all those who care about making the world a healthier place have reason to be grateful.

PAUL FARMER

ACKNOWLEDGMENTS

"AUTHOR" IS THE ACCEPTED TERM for my role in the production of this book, but it is not a completely accurate one. Quite often, I served simply as the compiler of stories, facts, figures, plans, and dreams lived and chronicled by many others, most of whom are heroes of the Indiana–Moi partnership and this book.

Understanding that I am inevitably going to forget to mention someone whose contribution was critical, it is imperative that I thank for their contributions of time, insight, information, and advice to making this book better: Joe Mamlin, Bob Einterz, Haroun Mengech, Sylvester Kimaiyo, Ellen Quigley, Lea Anne Einterz, Sarah Ellen Mamlin, Adrian Gardner, Daniel Ochieng, Michael Reece, Dee Mortensen, Nick Arena, David Bryden, Scott Pegg, Bob White, Allen Moore, Bill Quigley, Jim Greene, Kristi Tabaj, Ron Pettigrew, Becca Graffis, and Susan Moke. Chas Salmen, John Kratzer, Seth Einterz, and Francesca Cavallaro deserve special recognition for providing detailed and sensitive reporting on the amazing people that populate the AMPATH (Academic Model for Prevention and Treatment of HIV/AIDS) story. Along with the many generous individual and foundation donors mentioned in this book, the special partnerships AMPATH has enjoyed with Abbott Fund and Eli Lilly and Co. deserve acknowledgment and thanks.

My understanding of the AIDS crisis and the activism confronting it was helped immeasurably by reading and referring to Greg Behrman's *The Invisible People: How the U.S. Has Slept through the Global AIDS Pandemic, the Greatest Humanitarian Catastrophe of Our Time*; Derek Hodel's *At the Crossroads: A Study of Federal HIV/AIDS Advocacy*, a report for the Ford Foundation; and Stephanie Nolen's *28: Stories of AIDS in Africa*.

Any success that this book achieves in capturing the magic of the Indiana–Moi partnership is due to the efforts of many. Any errors or omissions are my fault alone.

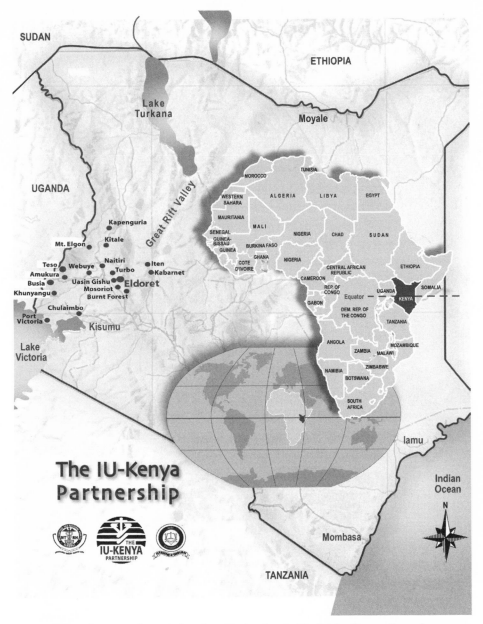

Map showing clinical sites for the Academic Model for Prevention of HIV/AIDS (AMPATH) in western Kenya.

WALKING TOGETHER,
WALKING FAR

1

DANIEL

LATE ONE EVENING IN SEPTEMBER of 2000, Dr. Joe Mamlin was making after-hours visits to some of his patients at Moi Teaching and Referral Hospital in Eldoret, Kenya. The wards he walked through were made up of several open rooms with a half-dozen small cot-like beds, most of which contained two patients lying with each one's head to the feet of his bed partner. Except for the dimly lit central corridor, the wards were completely dark. Mosquitoes and flies swarmed on the patients in the equatorial night.

Wards at Moi Hospital were organized into three bays on each side of the corridor, with six to eight beds in each bay. Bay 3 was farthest from the nursing station and closest to the stench from the perpetually clogged and broken flush toilets. Partly because many of the HIV patients also had highly contagious tuberculosis, they were all placed back in this forsaken area the Kenyan medical students had nicknamed "Bosnia." Bay 3's patients were mostly young people, ages eighteen to thirty-five. Most were parents of young children. All were expected to die within a few weeks.

This grim scene in the western highlands of Kenya was being replicated throughout Africa. By this time in 2000, the United Nations was estimating that 23 million people on the continent were infected with HIV. That year, 2.4 million Africans died from the disease and nearly 4 million were newly infected. In many parts of Africa, entire villages had been so ravaged by AIDS that they were populated almost entirely by old people and orphaned children.

When Mamlin arrived in Kenya three months before, the six-ty-six-year-old physician was looking to put the finishing touches on a career that had made him something of a local legend in Indianapolis. As a professor of medicine at Indiana University and as chief of medicine at Indianapolis's Wishard Memorial Hospital, Mamlin had spearheaded the creation of a groundbreaking neighborhood-centered health-care system for the poor. Before that, he had spent several years as a Peace Corps volunteer physician in Afghanistan with his wife, Sarah Ellen, and their three children, bringing up a new medical school in Jalalabad and treating patients under brutal conditions.

White-haired, well over six feet tall, and a lifelong student of philosophy, Mamlin is described by his colleague Dr. Bob Einterz as an "LBJ-type" figure. "Joe has had this mystique about him from the time he was chief resident at Wishard," Einterz says. "It comes from his combination of insatiable optimism, an enormous capacity to believe he is right, and the quintessential silver tongue—a remarkable ability to persuade others that his vision is the correct one."

Mamlin was no stranger to Kenya. In 1992 and 1993, he had served a term as the field director of Indiana University's partnership with Moi University School of Medicine. In the summer of 2000, when Mamlin retired from his Indiana duties, he and Sarah Ellen agreed that another year or two in Kenya would be the perfect springboard to full-time retirement.

But things had changed since Mamlin was last in Africa. Eight years before, he might have seen about eighty patients die on these hospital wards each year, most of them elderly. That many were dying each month now, and the dead patients were much younger. Mamlin's immediate predecessor as Indiana team leader in Eldoret was the young pediatrician and internist John Sidle, who had arrived in Kenya two years earlier full of enthusiasm for his African experience. Like the iconic figure of the worn-out Father Time at the end of each year, Sidle departed Kenya in bad shape. Devastated by the daily ordeal of watching his AIDS patients die, and frustrated by his inability to prescribe the drugs to treat them, Sidle was depressed and struggling with alcohol addiction. Even though Sidle had been one of Indiana's most successful team leaders in Eldoret, he left vowing never to return to Africa.

After just a few weeks back in Kenya, Mamlin knew how Sidle felt. "I find this to be the most difficult task of my entire career," he admitted. "It is easy to sit in a conference room and say it is not wise to provide treatment here. But it's a lot harder to be here and look into these people's eyes and not be doing anything." Einterz recalls those days as the only ones he ever knew Mamlin to be without optimism. The leader of Indiana's medical community was "in anguish," Einterz says.

That evening, Mamlin turned out of the lit corridor and into the darkened Bay 3. As his eyes adjusted, he recognized Moi University medical student Bernard Olayo sitting by one of the beds, spoon-feeding a gaunt young man whom Mamlin did not recognize. It was long past the hour when medical students usually left the hospital, so Mamlin asked why Olayo was there. Olayo gestured toward the patient he was feeding, and introduced Joe Mamlin to his friend and classmate, fifth-year medical student Daniel Ochieng.

❈

Daniel Ochieng grew up in the western Kenya village of Siaya near the city of Kisumu. His father, a schoolteacher, died when Daniel was just five years old, so his mother, Leonida, raised Daniel and his younger sister alone on their small farm. "When I was in primary school, I wanted to be a teacher, because in the village, the teachers were revered and were the only ones with a consistent income," Ochieng remembers. But when he began attending secondary school, Ochieng discovered he had a talent for the sciences. During his final year, he scored well enough on the nationwide medicine exam, a challenging combination of science, math, and language, to earn one of the coveted 150 medical school spots open to Kenyan students each year. Ochieng became the first person in his family to attend university.

"I was a social person, vocal in advocacy for student rights," Ochieng says. But during his fourth year as a medical student, both Ochieng's political advocacy and his plans to become a surgeon began to be affected by his deteriorating health. He started having chest pains and losing weight. He struggled to fight off repeated infections, including painful oral thrush, which coated his mouth and throat with a white cottony substance. Ultimately he was diagnosed with tuberculosis and hospitalized, where a test confirmed that he was HIV-positive.

As a medical student, Ochieng knew enough to be scared. "When we were doing rounds at the hospital, if one of the patients was HIV-positive, you knew they were definitely going to die," he said. Ochieng did not tell his family about his diagnosis, but he realized his professors and fellow medical students could likely guess his disease from his marked weight loss, constant diarrhea, and inability to fight off infections. Caroline Kosgei, one of his university classmates, remembers seeing Ochieng brought out of the student hostel in a wheelchair on his way to be admitted to the hospital across the street. "He was so wasted, it was horrible," she says. "We all went back to our rooms to cry."

Mamlin later described the Ochieng he saw that night, who had lost a third of his body weight until he was a mere 72 pounds, as a "breathing skeleton." Physicians consider HIV to have progressed to full-blown AIDS when a patient's CD4 count, a measure of the white blood cells per microliter of blood, drops to less than 200. Ochieng's CD4 count was 34. Ochieng's worried mother rushed to Eldoret to stay at his bedside. He did not tell his mother he was HIV-positive, but Ochieng knew enough about the medical reality to make it difficult to show any optimism. "I knew I would die if I did not get help," he said.

But even four years of African medical school had not given Ochieng much of a clue about what that help could be. Since no patient on the wards of Moi Teaching and Referral Hospital had ever been treated with antiretroviral drugs, Ochieng's clinical training never involved the regimen that had been proven to save the lives of HIV-positive patients.

In the fall of 2000, antiretroviral therapy for HIV/AIDS was working wonders in the United States and the western world. But the conventional wisdom shared by global health agencies, funders, and governments was that treatment in Africa was impossible. The $500-plus per month cost of the drugs was prohibitive for patients and governments in poor countries, where as much as half the population struggled to survive on less than $1 per day. The lack of functioning health systems in many African communities seemed to make it impossible to administer the exacting antiretroviral drug regimen, which must be followed every day of the patient's life.

In 2001, Andrew Natsios, the Bush administration's chief of the U.S. Agency for International Development (USAID), would tell the House International Relations Committee that it was impossible to provide antiretroviral drug treatment to the millions of Africans infected with HIV. Although Natsios was widely criticized for his statement that Africans' inability to tell "Western time" prevented them from being able to adhere to the antiretroviral regimen, others expressed more carefully worded concerns to justify the fact that virtually no Africans infected with HIV were being given antiretroviral drugs (ARVs).

For example, Julian Lambert, senior Africa AIDS specialist with Britain's Department for International Development, wrote in late 2000 in praise of the success of ARVs in the West. "However," Lambert wrote, "the treatment is currently much too expensive to be made widely available in developing countries, and would also require more effective health systems to support patients in following the drug regimes in order to prevent the development of resistance and mutation of the virus."

Lambert's view reflected the global health consensus that treatment in Africa would be so haphazard that it would actually worsen the pandemic by creating drug-resistant strains of HIV. As the twentieth century came to a close, the word had come down in no uncertain terms: In Africa, it was better to focus anti-AIDS efforts on prevention alone. Those already infected, including Daniel Ochieng, would be left to die.

※

In his few short weeks back in Kenya, Joe Mamlin had already seen dozens of young Kenyan men and women infected with AIDS waste away and die. Mamlin realized that it shouldn't have mattered that this particular patient, too weak to raise his arms to feed himself, was a medical student. But it did matter. Something about Daniel Ochieng lying next to another patient in the same bed, waiting for death in the dark of Bay 3, challenged all of the well-settled reasons why HIV/AIDS was not being treated in Africa.

Shaken by his encounter with Ochieng, Mamlin left the hospital that night and walked slowly to the house Indiana University rented a half mile away. By the time he reached his computer and logged on to the slow dial-up connection to the internet, Mamlin had made up his mind. He began to compose an e-mail to Einterz, the Indianapolis-based director of the Indiana–Moi partnership.

By nearly any measure, that partnership was already a remarkable success story. Since 1989, hundreds of Indiana University medical students, residents, and faculty members had come to Eldoret as part of the program, with at least one full-time Indiana faculty member always on-site for at least a one-year term. Dozens of Kenyan faculty members and students, most on full fellowships or scholarships, had traveled to Indianapolis for advanced training. Praise for the program flowed in from faculty, students, and international relations experts from both countries. Impoverished Kenyans had been treated; technical and cultural information had been exchanged. Collaborative research had been conducted. Current and future generations of U.S. and Kenyan doctors had forged cross-cultural relationships that enriched both communities.

Mamlin noted all that in his message to Einterz. But he also wrote that it might be time to put an end to the program. With Kenyans like Ochieng dying by the hundreds each week, the partnership simply could not continue on as before. Indiana University must fully engage in the struggle against HIV/AIDS, Mamlin insisted, or it should fold its tents and go home. Personally, he had no intention of standing by and watching an entire generation of Kenyans die, even from a disease that was considered too expensive and difficult to treat in Africa.

Copies remain of some of Mamlin's e-mail messages from that time, in particular one September exchange that began with a message to Dr. Joe Wheat, an infectious diseases specialist at

Indiana University School of Medicine. "Joe, I would like for you to consider helping me with a tough problem," Mamlin began, and then explained Daniel Ochieng's situation.

"I have seen more HIV in these three months I have been here than all the docs in Indiana combined," Mamlin wrote. "Yet I have seen no one treated for HIV—we treat the TB, typhoid, pneumonias, etc. and let the retrovirus do its thing—which it does relentlessly." Mamlin wanted to make Ochieng the first HIV patient to be treated with antiretrovirals in the history of the Indiana–Moi partnership and the public wards of Moi Hospital. He asked for Wheat's help in guiding the regimen and finding the money to do it.

Mamlin shared this request with several of his Indiana colleagues. The reaction was mixed. John Sidle had helped Ochieng with food and medicine while Sidle was in Kenya. "I like Daniel and I would like to help him," Sidle wrote in reply to Mamlin's message, offering to try to find some donated medicines for Ochieng. But Sidle, fresh from Africa, knew well the challenges Indiana would face in treating a single patient in a community and country where millions were dying untreated. "The reality is that he [Daniel] is only one of what will probably be many cases among the faculty and medical students over the next few years," Sidle wrote. "Where do we draw the line and how do we presume to choose who does or does not get the few medicines we have? [Also,] compliance is so important that unless we can get a steady supply this is going to be difficult."

As the administrator of the program back in Indiana, Einterz might have been expected to raise a red flag in front of Mamlin's impulse. Even if successful, treating Daniel Ochieng was a lifetime financial commitment for a program that had no revenue to draw from. And there was no way to answer Sidle's question of how Indiana–Moi would respond to the next Kenyan student—or physician—who began fading from AIDS. If unsuccessful, the program's prestige within the United States and Kenya would be damaged for a foolish effort to defy the accepted protocol for responding to AIDS in Africa. But less than an hour after Sidle expressed his concerns, Einterz responded with his own argument for treating Daniel Ochieng. "The anguish of watching a colleague die of a treatable illness makes us try to do something—to do nothing forsakes hope," he wrote. "Yes, the question is where do we draw the line but perhaps, in our asking, we will find that we should never draw it."

Einterz empathized with the anguish of his colleagues as they watched Kenyans die from AIDS while their HIV/AIDS patients in the United States were almost always successfully treated. When Einterz served as the program's first Kenya-based team leader in 1991, a meningitis epidemic broke out. "Fifteen people would come into the hospital during the day with meningitis, and all would be dead the next morning," he recalls. "They could be treated with simple penicillin, but the hospital had run out and no one could afford to buy more." A lifesaving daily dose of penicillin cost about $2.

Einterz remembers walking to the Eldoret post office to make a phone call to Mamlin and their fellow Indiana–Moi founder Dr. Charlie Kelley. "When we went to Kenya, we made the commitment that we were going to work within the Kenyan system and only do what we could do within the system," Einterz recalls now. "We were not going to inject money into the system. The clash is between relief and development, of course. We knew that paying for a bunch of things could be detrimental for development because we were providing the fish rather than teaching the Kenyans to fish. The first test of that theory was the meningitis epidemic, and we immediately realized that at some point, we could not confine ourselves to working within the existing system."

Einterz used his own money to purchase the penicillin. "When he wanted to treat Daniel, Joe was breaking all of our rules," Einterz says. "But I understood completely, because I did the same thing. I just couldn't stand by and watch all those people dying needless deaths."

Nearly a decade later and in the face of an epidemic like no other the world has ever seen, Mamlin couldn't either. He continued writing long messages back to Indiana, making his case for treating Ochieng. "This medical faculty [in Kenya] needs to see an example of something other than doom and gloom—which is all around us. It is also important that they see one of their peers taking his 'head out of the sand' and facing reality with this plague. This stigma thing is overwhelming here. This young man is a step in the right direction toward seeing this as a disease with a treatment rather than a 'curse' which is to be shunned."

"We may be opening Pandora's box—but no less so than when we decided to come here in the first place," he wrote. Mamlin's message closed with a quote from theologian Reinhold Niebuhr: "Nothing worth doing is completed in our lifetime; we must be saved by hope."

Within two weeks of these cross-continental discussions, the infectious disease department of Indiana University School of Medicine agreed to send $10,000 to Kenya to provide for a year and a half of treatment for Ochieng. Eventually, Mamlin would stretch that donation by using a supply of pills cobbled together back in Indiana, mostly from those left over by American HIV patients when they changed to new drug regimens.

Mamlin immediately started Ochieng on the drugs. For a month, Ochieng was still too weak to leave his bed. Every morning, he would wake to the sound of a rickety aluminum hospital cart taking away the bodies of his fellow Bay 3 patients who had died in the night. But soon the antiretrovirals' nearly magical power—so potent it is widely described as the "Lazarus effect"— took hold in Ochieng. Mamlin remembers walking between hospital wards one day and noticing a patient sitting on the grass soaking in the sun. It was Ochieng. It was then, Mamlin said, that he knew the young man would survive. In one of the most miraculous recoveries that Mamlin had ever witnessed in over forty years of practicing medicine, Daniel Ochieng walked out of Moi Teaching and Referral Hospital six weeks after receiving his first dose of antiretroviral medicine. Ochieng is certain he was the only patient from his time in Bay 3 to leave the hospital alive.

For a year, Ochieng remained the only Indiana–Moi patient receiving antiretrovirals. But his dramatic recovery made it even more difficult for Mamlin and other Indiana–Moi physicians to stand by and watch other AIDS patients die without treatment. "Daniel's recovery was the first hope that any of us saw in Kenya," Einterz said. The cross-continental calls, e-mails, and visits continued, evoking Ochieng's successful recovery and questioning the idea that HIV/AIDS could not be treated in sub-Saharan Africa.

As Ochieng continued to regain strength, Mamlin wrote back to Indiana. "At the end of the day, IU will, to a large extent, be judged by the energy and wisdom we bring into the 'unappreciated' chaos thrust upon us by AIDS . . . Without the magic bullet of a vaccine, one is left with the unbelievable complexity of prevention strategies, education, and unaffordable (and probably unmanageable) treatment efforts. What does one do? Just fold our hands and walk away? Continue the cover-up conspiracy and just 'do' the wards and shut up? Or, is there really something we can do—regardless of how small—that is aimed in the right direction? Something that gives evidence by our role model that we SEE this damn thing and we mean to fight back?"

Widespread HIV/AIDS treatment was still being described, even by the optimistic Mamlin, as "unaffordable" and "probably unmanageable." But a small academic partnership was already being transformed into a program that would become a globally acclaimed success story and one of the models for confronting history's most deadly pandemic.

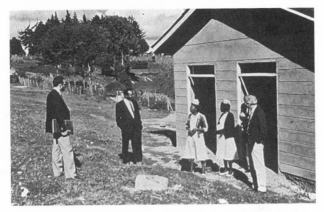

Figure 1. Indiana University's first visit to Eldoret in 1988. Dr. Bob Einterz and Dr. Haroun Mengech are on the left, Dr. Joe Mamlin on the extreme right.
PHOTO BY CHARLIE KELLEY.

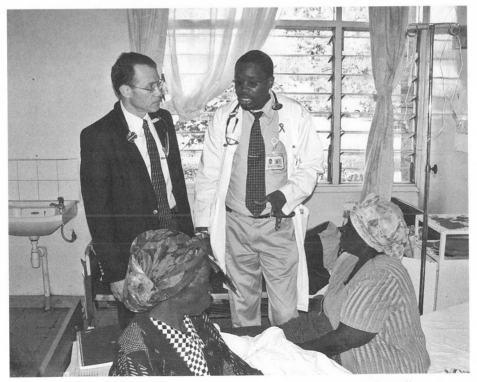

Figure 2. Indiana University's Dr. Bob Einterz consults with Kenyan colleague Dr. Paul Muganda while examining patients at Moi Teaching and Referral Hospital.
PHOTO BY SHAWN WOODIN.

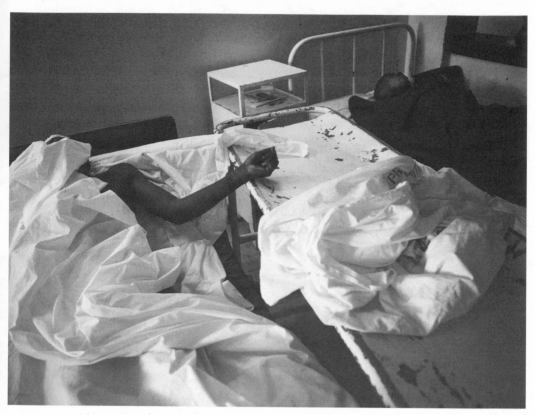

Figure 3. Before Moi and Indiana physicians began providing antiretroviral treatment for HIV/AIDS, patients diagnosed with HIV at Moi Teaching and Referral Hospital rarely left the hospital alive. In 2000, 2.4 million Africans died from the disease, as HIV treatment was virtually nonexistent on the continent.

Photo by Tyagan Miller.

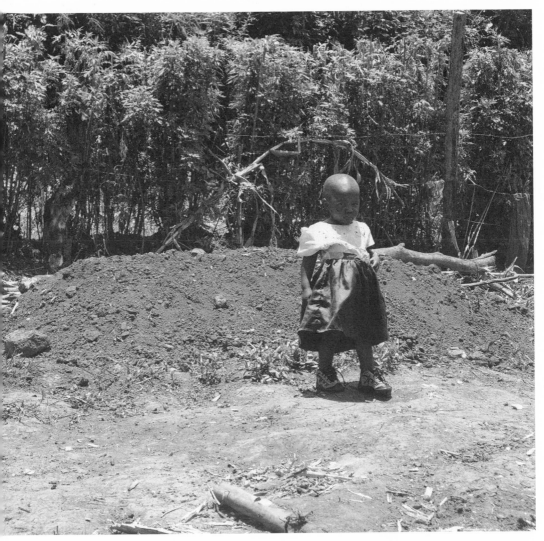

Figure 4. By 2007, an estimated 12 million African children had been orphaned by HIV/AIDS, including this little Kenyan girl posing in front of her mother's grave.

PHOTO BY JOE MAMLIN.

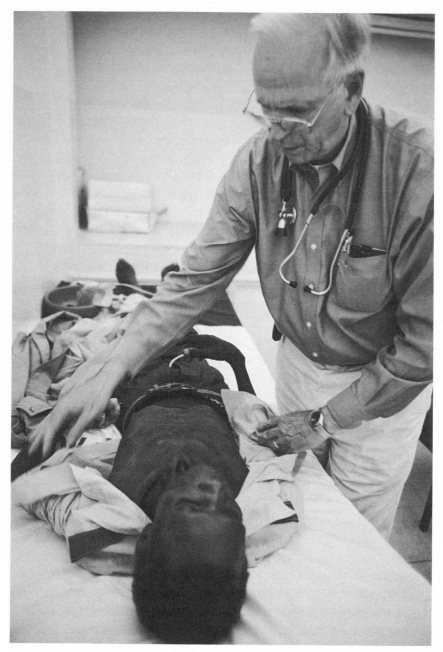

Figure 5. Indiana University's Dr. Joe Mamlin examines a patient severely wasted from AIDS.

Photo by Tyagan Miller.

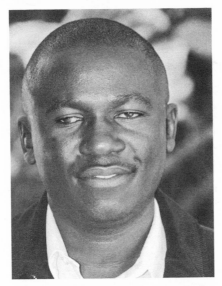

Figure 6. In late 2000, Moi University School of Medicine student Daniel Ochieng became the first HIV-positive person to be treated by what would become AMPATH, the Academic Model for Prevention and Treatment of HIV/AIDS.
PHOTO BY FRAN QUIGLEY.

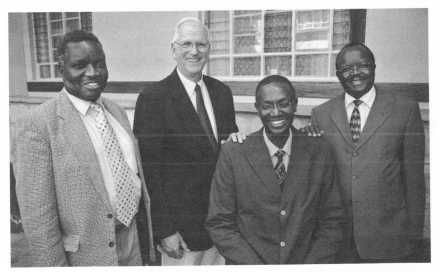

Figure 7. From left to right, Moi University School of Medicine dean Dr. Fabian Esamai, Indiana University field director Dr. Joe Mamlin, AMPATH program manager Dr. Sylvester Kimaiyo, and Moi Teaching and Referral Hospital director Dr. Haroun Mengech.
PHOTO BY TYAGAN MILLER.

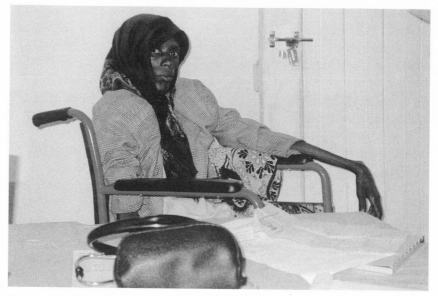

Figure 8. Before treatment was widely available, patients with advanced AIDS, like this severely wasted woman, often did not come to AMPATH clinics until it was too late.
PHOTO BY FRAN QUIGLEY.

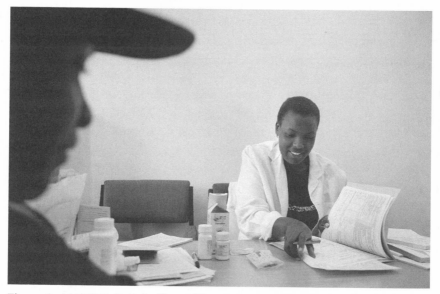

Figure 9. AMPATH clinical officer Lillian Boit reviews a patient's treatment record at the rural Mosoriot clinic. By the end of 2007, AMPATH was treating over 50,000 HIV-positive patients at 18 clinical sites throughout western Kenya.
WORLD HEALTH ORGANIZATION/EVELYN HOCKSTEIN.

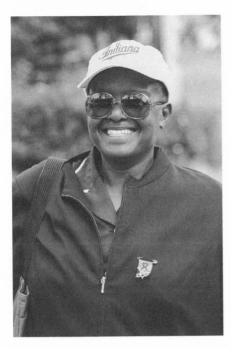

Figures 10 and 11. Mosoriot clinic director and nurse Irene Kalamai helped AMPATH partner with traditional Kenyan birth attendants to provide education and treatment that helps block transmission of the virus from HIV-positive mothers to their babies.

PHOTOS BY FRAN QUIGLEY.

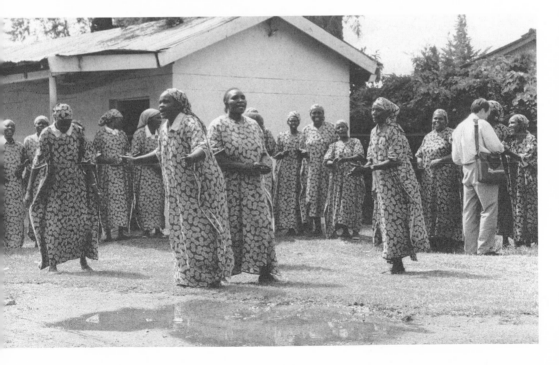

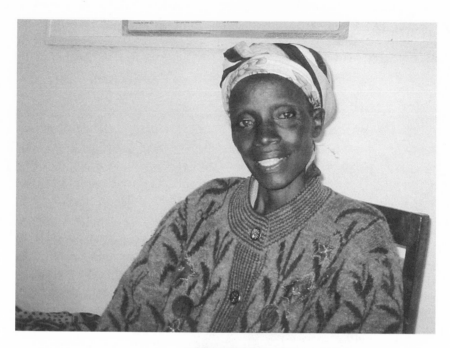

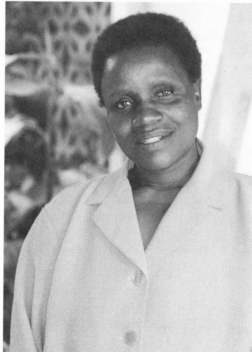

Figures 12 and 13. AMPATH patient Salina Rotich before and after receiving nutrition support to supplement her antiretroviral treatment.

First photo by Joe Mamlin.
Second photo by Fran Quigley.

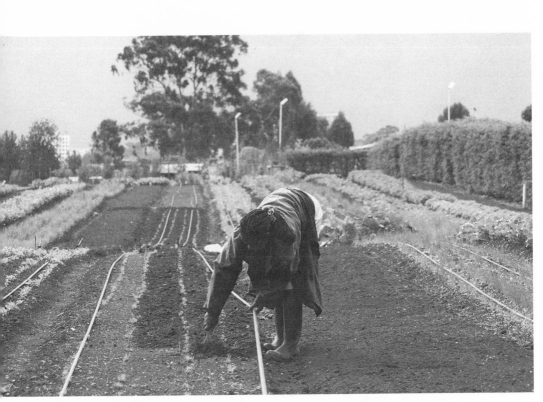

Figure 14. AMPATH's high-production farms yield vegetables and dairy products that, supplemented with UN World Food Program donations, feed 30,000 persons each week.

PHOTO BY FRAN QUIGLEY.

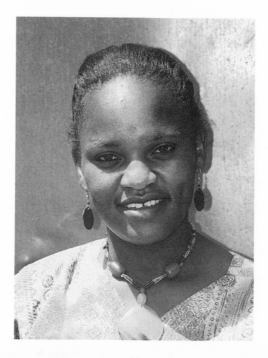

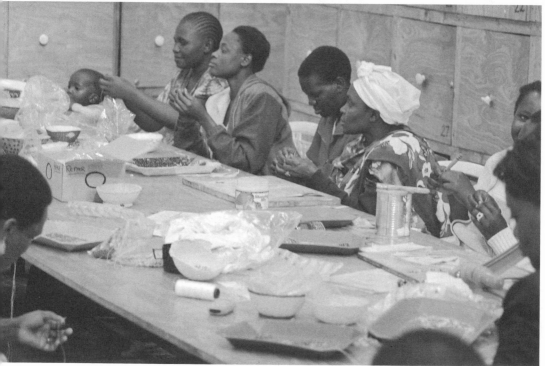

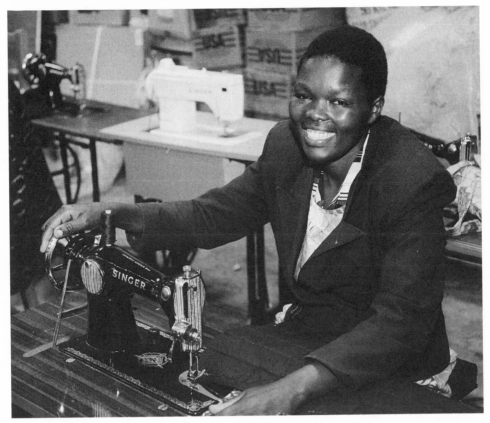

Figures 15, 16, and 17: AMPATH patient (top left) Evelyne Njoki's success at making and selling jewelry to support herself and her baby inspired the creation of the Imani Workshops, which has trained and employed thousands of HIV-positive artisans in making jewelry, crafts, and clothing for sale in Kenya and the United States.

FIRST TWO PHOTOS BY FRAN QUIGLEY. THIRD PHOTO BY TYAGAN MILLER.

BIRTH OF A PARTNERSHIP

IN 1985, THE *JOURNAL OF THE AMERICAN MEDICAL ASSOCIATION* published a list of more than seventy organizations that provided health services internationally. Twenty-nine-year-old Bob Einterz, fresh from a stint as chief resident physician at Indianapolis's Wishard Hospital, and in his first year as a faculty member at Indiana University School of Medicine, sat down and typed letters to each organization, offering to serve as a volunteer doctor for a year.

He received just one positive answer, from Minnesota International Health Volunteers. So Einterz signed up with the Minnesota group, who sent Einterz, his wife Lea Anne, and their two young boys to Croix Fer, Haiti, a dusty, desperately poor community just a few kilometers west of the border with the Dominican Republic.

In Haiti, Einterz saw patients at a clinic every day, and every Tuesday he walked in the blistering heat to one of the remote villages to announce that he would be giving immunizations the next day. The following day, Einterz, a village health worker, and a nurse would repeat the same walk, carrying a cold pack of vaccines. Children and mothers would line up, usually outside the dilapidated village church, where Einterz would direct a make-shift clinic the rest of the day.

Before one of the Tuesday announcement visits, Einterz was able to obtain a jeep from the Haitian Ministry of Health to drive up a rugged mountain road to that week's temporary village clinic location. He invited Lea Anne to come along and bring their boys, Robbie, only two years old, and baby Zach, who was less than a year. On their way home, a sudden rainstorm turned the dirt road into a river of mud, and the jeep became hopelessly stuck. With no food or water, they had no choice but to walk down the mountain. Bob had to tie his sandals to his feet with twine to keep them from being sucked off in the mud, and Robbie was carried down the mountain on the back of a mule guided by Pierre, the husband of the chief clinic nurse. By the time they finally reached the bottom of the mountain, it was well after dark.

During most of their year in Croix Fer, the Einterz family had no car, no electricity, and no running water. After putting the boys to bed in their tin-roofed home with no glass or screens on the windows, Bob and Lea Anne would play Scrabble by the light of a kerosene lantern. When the game ended, they turned off the lantern and quickly jumped into bed under the mosquito netting before the bats flew in through the windows.

"That year was a huge baptism for me," Einterz says. "I learned firsthand about the concept of primary health care, a physician's role in the community, and the role of economics and culture in health care. We worked on income generation, family planning, and creating mothers' groups. I learned about the critically important role of women in development. Overall, the experience working side-by-side in the community taught me both about the complexity of delivering quality public health and about the importance of community to tackle these problems.

"These were things not covered in med school, and they hit me in the face in rural Haiti."

But Einterz's background had prepared him unusually well to face challenges to conventional wisdom. By the time Einterz entered junior high school, his father, Frank, a manager of food-processing plants, and his mother, Cora, had moved their ever-growing family several times, first within New York State, then to St. Joseph, Michigan, and finally to Indianapolis. Frank chaired heated nightly discussions around the dinner table, and lectured the thirteen children on the virtues of the Stoic philosophers, including Epictetus and Marcus Aurelius, along with the basics of Jesuit and Franciscan theology. It was a socially conservative and intellectually demanding Roman Catholic upbringing that emphasized the principle that with privilege comes responsibility. All of the children were encouraged to speak their mind—and to be prepared to defend themselves from the inevitable challenges launched by siblings or parents.

Einterz's elder siblings Frank Jr. and Ellen both joined the Peace Corps and headed to Africa, Frank to Kenya and Ellen to Niger. Einterz's first exposure to Eldoret came in 1977 when he was visiting his brother. Einterz had wanted to be a doctor since he was a child. "I had a pretty romantic view of what a physician was," he says. "But for me, the profession seemed right. I never enjoyed playing make-believe as a kid, and I still don't understand why anyone would read a fantasy novel instead of a biography." A girl Einterz dated in high school wrote him an e-mail more than thirty years later recalling that he had pledged even as a teenager to do work in Africa.

The rigors of a difficult premed and medical school academic regimen suited Einterz's ambitious and serious nature. At Indianapolis North Central High and at male-only Wabash College in rural Crawfordsville, Indiana, Einterz played football and was on the wrestling and track teams. But he was conspicuously absent from parties and trips to the movies, and rarely even watched television. "I was a pretty damn intense student," he says. "Plus, I have always been something of a social introvert—I still struggle with small talk." During his year as chief resident at Wishard Hospital, Einterz worked 330 consecutive days without a day off, including the day Lea Anne gave birth to their firstborn, Robert Jr.

Einterz had always idolized his older brother, and he was close to his older sister, who taught him to read while Einterz was still a preschooler, so he wanted to follow in their footsteps of international service. "Dad always drove home the point that our Catholic faith demands we make the most of the gifts we have been given," he says. "At its core, being a physician is about helping others, so I think I took that to heart."

After Haiti, Einterz returned to the Indiana faculty and began working to create an opportunity for other young physicians to get the same international experience he had. He talked with Joe Mamlin, his boss in the medical school's Division of General Internal Medicine, about how Indiana University could create that opportunity. "It was Joe who felt so strongly that the best way to do this was to link with another medical school," Einterz says.

🌿

Mamlin, it turned out, had some unfinished business of his own in the developing world. In 1965, two decades earlier, he had been at the same stage of his career as Einterz was when he sent out his seventy letters: completing his own tenure as chief resident at Marion County General Hospital, whose name would soon be changed to Wishard. Mamlin traveled back to his home state of North Carolina to interview for what he describes now as a "dream fellowship" in cardiology at Duke University. At Duke, he would have been able to pursue a medical specialty he found fascinating, and enjoy a comfortable faculty position to boot. But on his way back to Indiana from the Duke interview, Mamlin stopped in Washington, D.C., and talked with the Peace Corps about starting a medical school in Jalalabad, Afghanistan. To counter Duke's exciting cardiology fellowship offer, the Peace Corps promised Mamlin $75 a month and a bicycle.

Mamlin grew up in Asheville, North Carolina, as the third of four children born to a Jewish father, who sold shoes at a store called The Bootery, and a Southern Baptist mother whose schooling stopped at third grade. "Asheville was quite stratified then," Mamlin's childhood friend Jim Greene recalls. "The Mamlins lived in West Asheville, and that was definitely the other side of the tracks." Joe Mamlin remembers welfare assistance, in the form of food and some money, occasionally being delivered to the family home.

From junior high onward, the Mamlin children were expected to earn money for their own clothes and other expenses. Joe

Mamlin set up pins in a bowling alley, worked as a soda jerk, and sold clothes at the local JCPenney store. "We did not have any academic culture in our house, and our parents did not give us any money for college education," he says. "But they gave us exactly what we needed for life—the understanding of what it was like to do hard work. Whenever we left the house, our mother would say to us, 'Remember you are a Mamlin.' That inculcated a sense of self that is invaluable."

No one in the family was too concerned when Joe did not finish high school. After all, he was already working, which was the most important thing for a Mamlin. Then one day a customer buying children's clothes from Mamlin at the Asheville JCPenney offered to introduce him to her husband, who was the president of Mars Hill College, a junior college in the Blue Ridge Mountains just north of Asheville. The college president gave Mamlin a one-semester trial admission.

Suddenly, Mamlin discovered life as a student. At Mars Hill, he met and began dating his future wife, Sarah Ellen Dozier, the daughter of a third-generation Baptist missionary, who had spent most of her childhood in Japan. Already an active youth member of the First Baptist Church in Asheville, Mamlin began preparing for a career in the ministry. While working as a lumberjack in Oregon the summer after his first year of college, he did some preaching at a little mountain church.

But while hitchhiking home to North Carolina from that summer job, Mamlin was severely injured when the car he was riding in collided head-on with a truck. Lying flat on his back in traction for six weeks in a New Mexico hospital, his hip broken and his face and arms deeply cut in multiple places, he got to see the world of medicine up close for the first time.

Mamlin had been dismayed by his experience working with the senior preacher near the lumberjack camp in Oregon. "He had the superficiality of a TV evangelist, speaking from underlined Bible passages that of course told us all that we needed to know about what is right," Mamlin says. At the same time, Mamlin had been energized by the vigorous communal work of logging. "I concluded that maybe the best way to be of value in this world is to work and not talk," he says. After he recovered and returned to school, Mamlin switched his major to premed, transferred to Wake Forest University, and promptly got straight As for the first time in his life.

There was no money for medical school, though, so Mamlin's goal to become a doctor seemed remote. Then he was nominated to compete for one of the eight scholarships to Wake Forest's medical school being offered by North Carolina tobacco heir R. J. Reynolds, Jr. Mamlin and the other would-be Reynolds scholars were invited to a cocktail reception and dinner at a country club. Mamlin, who had never been to a country club before and was a Baptist teetotaler, was uncomfortable with the before-dinner chatter. Instead of mingling, he ended up deep in conversation with an older man who had an obvious breathing problem. When they sat down to dinner, Mamlin discovered that the man he had befriended was R. J. Reynolds, Jr., himself. Mamlin got the very first scholarship awarded.

The Reynolds scholarship paid for all of Mamlin's medical school costs at Wake Forest and for two years of residency at Marion County General Hospital, soon to be Wishard. "I graduated without a penny of debt," he says. "Which made it possible for Sarah Ellen and me to reach for the grand offer of $75 a month and a bicycle in Jalalabad."

By then, the Mamlins had three young children—not exactly a typical Peace Corps volunteer profile. And Afghanistan was a mystery to both the Mamlins and their family and friends, who often asked what part of Africa they would be moving to. But Sarah Ellen Mamlin, who had lived with her missionary parents in Japan before and after World War II and witnessed the Pearl Harbor bombings from the second story of a home in Honolulu, was not concerned. "When Joe and I were in college together, we thought we were likely going to be overseas missionaries," she says. "I never thought I would spend my whole life in the United States."

In Afghanistan, Mamlin labored to nurture the fledgling Nangarhar University School of Medicine in a setting more deprived than he could have imagined. In a May 1967 letter to his Peace Corps superiors, Mamlin described the scene: "As I write this, the majority of the patients in the hospital have no drugs available—

they are weeks overdue—no x-ray all year, no blood bank, not a single student or doctor has the equipment to do a simple physical exam, and no student has a textbook or dictionary, to name a few have-nots." The Afghan patients and their families understood the grim prospects this scarcity foretold. "When a patient is acutely ill, the family does not even give us a chance," Mamlin wrote. "They pick him up and carry him home because the taxi fare is only 40 to 60 afghanis (53 to 78 cents), but if he dies in the hospital, the taxi fare for a dead person is 2,000 to 3,000 afghanis ($25 to $40). None of these families can afford to let a relative die in the hospital."

Mamlin's own family was struggling with the punishing heat, which in Jalalabad exceeded 110 degrees daily in the summer months, and the children suffered from hepatitis and chronic diarrhea. For many years afterward, Sarah Ellen was too embarrassed to show slides of photos from their home there, because living on a dirt road frequented by dust-billowing trucks left the house in a perpetual state of grime. But they persevered, escaping to Kabul during the worst weeks of summer while Mamlin translated his medical lectures into Pashto to create the only modern medical text available in his students' language.

Back in Jalalabad, Mamlin held nightly seminars at his home and bought drugs and equipment with funds donated by his colleagues back in Indiana. In a letter home thanking one of the donors, Mamlin wrote, "I try to choose the patients where we have some hope. The results have been rewarding. Not only have we saved some lives, but it points out to the students and doctors the value of the individual. Last week I talked a family out of taking their fourteen-year-old son home who had hookworm and a temperature of 105 degrees from typhoid. But when I came in the next morning he was gone. The family was afraid we were going to poison him. I became so angry that I sent one of our residents out to find the boy. Three hours later he found him on the ground in the corner of a windowless room . . . left to die. My resident told me he had to crawl on the ground on his hands and knees until he felt the body because there was no light in the room. He brought him back and with the money from the fund, we bought five units of blood and Chloramphenicol [an antibiotic] from Kabul. This boy is now eating us out of house and home, is afebrile [without fever] and very much alive."

As Haiti would be for Einterz two decades later, Afghanistan was a life-changing experience for Mamlin. "I fell in love with medical education in the context of a developing country," he says. "That fit my genome. My love of philosophy, theology, my love of guesswork all came into play. Peace Corps taught me about counterparts: rather than go to a developing country to be a hero, empower a hero in that culture. And the experience taught me about the multiplier effect—training forty students to be effective doctors has more payoff than anything I could do on my own."

So when a limousine pulled up in front of his house in Jalalabad and a royal guard emerged to say that Mamlin's presence was urgently needed to care for the ill Queen Homaira Shah, Mamlin refused to go. Instead, he gave the guard the addresses of his Afghan counterparts and told him they were capable of providing excellent care to her highness. "If I went around them, it would have destroyed everything we were trying to accomplish," he says.

But Mamlin's efforts in Afghanistan did not lead to the long-term solution he was hoping for. His goal, expressed in multiple letters home to his colleagues in Indiana, was a medical school partnership that would address so many of the resource and expertise needs of the Afghan medical students and faculty physicians. "When I returned, I really felt I was going to hook Indiana University to Afghanistan on a school-to-school level," Mamlin says. "I worked on it for years. But then Afghanistan became Humpty Dumpty politically and I realized that I had lost it." After the Soviet invasion of 1979, all of the Afghan medical faculty whom Mamlin had trained fled to Pakistan, where they became refugees.

❀

Ten years later, and nearly twenty years after he left Afghanistan, Mamlin saw in Einterz hope for another chance at an international partnership for the Indiana University medical school.

Mamlin and Einterz brought into their discussions their fellow
Indiana faculty members Charlie Kelley, who had also spent time
teaching and treating patients in Afghanistan, and Dave Van Rek-
en, who had served as a missionary in Liberia. The four doctors
decided they should visit several medical schools in developing
countries and evaluate potential partners for Indiana University.

Einterz's large Catholic family provided an unexpected connection that allowed the four to raise the funds for the initial
trip. Einterz's younger sister Katey, then a student at Indianapolis North Central High, satisfied a social studies assignment in
part by reading aloud to the class excerpts of letters from Nigeria
sent home by her sister Ellen. Intrigued, Katey's teacher, Marty
Moore, asked to meet Ellen Einterz and then Bob Einterz, who
explained the ambitious plans for Indiana University to partner
with a medical school in the developing world. Moore had a small
family foundation and agreed to provide the seed money for the
Indiana physicians to visit and evaluate potential partners.

In November 1988, Einterz, Mamlin, Kelley, and Van Rek-
en left on a three-week tour to visit the Institute of Medicine
in Kathmandu, Nepal; Moi University in Eldoret, Kenya; and
the School of Medical Sciences at the University of Science and
Technology in Kumasi, Ghana. In Eldoret, then a city of about
250,000 people in western Kenya, they met at the downtown
Sirikwa Hotel with Dr. Haroun N. K. arap Mengech, the maverick
dean of a nonexistent medical school who was in the midst of
upsetting the medical establishment of Kenya.

Mengech was the middle child of nine siblings raised in the
Nandi district of the western Kenya highlands. His father moved
back and forth between positions as a teacher and local official
in the colonial and then postcolonial governments, before settling into a career as the pastor of a Pentecostal Assemblies of
God church. Mengech did well in his studies, but he was more
interested in returning to his agrarian roots than in following the
traditional Kenyan top-student path toward medical school. "I
grew up as Nandi with the cows and the goats, so I wanted to do
veterinary medicine," he says. But at the urging of the dean of
the University of Nairobi School of Medicine, then the only medical school in Kenya, Mengech agreed to learn how to treat hu-

mans. His first intention was to become a pediatrician, but those plans were derailed during his hospital internship. "I grew very attached to a few of the kids on the ward, and one of them died," he says. "It affected me very deeply, so I told myself if death is going to affect me this way, I'm not cut out for this."

At the suggestion of a professor, Mengech turned to psychiatry, then obtained postgraduate training in Scotland and joined the Nairobi medical school faculty. He recalls teaching his initial class, on memory and the human mind, to first-year students, and being struck by their intense engagement in the course. "I could not go ten minutes without them asking questions. They were lively and inquisitive and I really enjoyed teaching the class. But then a few years later I saw these same students in their clinical rotations, and they were like zombies. They had spent year after year being forced to simply memorize things, and they could no longer think for themselves."

A frustrated Mengech wrote several journal articles criticizing the old British lecture system for medical education. (About ten years earlier, Mamlin had complained similarly in a letter home from Afghanistan about students "stuck in a mire of memorization and regurgitation.") At the same time that Mengech's articles began circulating, Kenyan president Daniel arap Moi convened the Mackey Commission on education in Kenya. The commission recommended the creation of a second Kenyan medical school, to be located in Eldoret, and echoed Mengech's critiques of the medical education process. Mengech was asked to return home to western Kenya to lead this new school.

He said no. "I was very comfortable in Nairobi," he says now. "I had a busy practice, I was head of my department, and I was doing some research." Mengech was approached several times more before finally agreeing to take the position of dean, but only on his own terms. He demanded the right to create his own clearly defined curriculum, and insisted that a physical structure for the school be in place before he would admit the first student.

Mengech began to travel extensively to medical schools with community-based curricula, including McMaster University in Canada, Ben-Gurion University of the Negev in Israel, the University of Linköping in Sweden, and the University of Maastricht in the Netherlands. He concluded that a community-based experience and service (COBES) program would be the core of the new school's curriculum. The existing Kenyan model kept medical students away from the hospital for their entire first two years of schooling, but Mengech drafted plans to expose all medical students to some clinical education beginning with their first year. The clinical experience, just 20 percent of the course work for first-year students, would grow to 80 percent of the schedule for fourth-year students. "You don't expect a first-year medical student to examine a patient, of course, but you want them to relate the textbook problems to real people," Mengech says. "The patient's situation becomes the tutorial problem."

Mengech's curriculum plan met resistance within the Kenyan Ministry of Education, and as the months passed after his appointment, he was also pushed to take on students before a building was constructed. Later, when asked if he felt pressure during this period, Mengech shrugs and smiles. "That was my agreement—no physical infrastructure, no students. Besides, I didn't ask for the job." It would be three full years between the time Mengech accepted the appointment of dean of the Moi University Faculty of Health Sciences and the admission of its first students. By then, Mengech had his building.

Mengech was already earning a reputation as a graceful navigator of the labyrinth of Kenyan officialdom, characterized too often by a frustrating mix of ethnic rivalries and corruption. (In Transparency International's 2008 global corruption rankings, Kenya tied for twentieth most corrupt nation in the world.) But Mengech nearly always emerged from the opaque system clutching a good result. Mamlin would later describe Mengech's ability to overcome bureaucratic barriers as part of the reason why Mengech was the Kenyan leader most responsible for the growth of the partnership. "Whether it is a container of medical supplies stuck in Customs, an employee's correct work permit being blocked, or the job of a nurse at a rural health clinic being threatened, Mengech is always able to clear it up," Mamlin says.

Mengech attributes that success to simple perseverance. "It is not the worst thing in life to tell me 'No,' or even to tell me to get the hell out of your office. That won't hurt me. So I'll go to anybody. I make an appointment. If they won't give me an appointment, I'll find out when they go to the office in the morning, get there before that, and wait for them."

When pushed, Mengech is willing to concede that his professional training helps the process, too. "You are forced to have patience in psychiatry. Solutions don't come quickly or easily. You can spend hour after hour with a patient with zero result. But you have to go back. That patience is important in this system."

Mengech eventually concluded that the district hospital in Eldoret, which was dirty and underfunded and kept no written patient records, was holding back the educational process for his medical students. He undertook to have the government redesignate the facility as a national referral hospital, a status that would provide more government funds and more autonomy. Mengech began a painstaking process of visiting the offices of the minister of health, the attorney general, and eventually the president of Kenya, quietly but persistently making his case. Ultimately, a decree changing the hospital's status was published in the official *Kenya Gazette* and became law, much to the surprise of many observers who had not noticed Mengech's efforts behind closed doors. "People asked me how it happened and I said I did not know," Mengech laughs. "I said, 'It's just government.'"

Mengech remembers first hearing about Indiana University's interest in partnering with Moi from a colleague in Nairobi, who told him, "These people from Indiana are looking for a partner, and they are interested in the wild ideas you have." Indeed they were. In a hotel room in Ghana at the end of their November 1988 tour, the Indiana physicians discussed which of the three schools they had visited would be the ideal partner. Citing Mengech's leadership and commitment to community-based education and care, along with the opportunity to get in on the ground floor of a brand-new institution, they agreed that Moi University was the right choice.

"WE ALL NEED TO BE DOING MORE"

AFTER THE MOI UNIVERSITY AND Indiana University medical schools formalized the decision to begin a partnership, Bob Einterz agreed to be the first Indiana faculty physician to spend a full year in Kenya. He was the first in an annual rotation of "team leaders" who practice medicine, teach at Moi University, and oversee Indiana students and residents. Bob, his wife Lea Anne, and their growing family of three boys arrived in Eldoret in July 1990, and soon settled into a house they rented from one Ibrahim Hussein, who happened to be a three-time winner of the Boston Marathon. They discovered that Eldoret's temperate climate and 7,000-foot altitude formed the cradle of Kenya's legendary running champions. In Eldoret, it was not unusual to bump into an Olympic gold medalist on the street or see a former world-record holder at the next table in a restaurant.

By the time Einterz arrived, Mengech had hired a dozen faculty members, and the first-ever Moi University medical school class, forty students strong, began their studies that fall. Six Indiana University medical students and residents spent time in Kenya that first year. Einterz especially enjoyed the experience of working in the rural health clinic in the Kosirai district of Mosoriot, a community that would become a critical part of the program's HIV outreach nearly twenty years later.

"I learned in Haiti that we could not make real change by confining ourselves to the four walls of the hospital or the examining room. The push toward the community began with the inception of the relationship with Moi," Einterz says. "'Community-based' was almost all that mattered to me." So Einterz's efforts that first year focused on championing the community-based education and service of COBES; for a full month he even lived without his family in spare quarters at the Mosoriot health center.

After a year, Einterz was followed by Charlie Kelley and then Joe Mamlin as team leaders for Indiana. In 1991, Diana Meneya and Gabriel Anabwani became the first Moi physicians to travel to Indiana. The partnership moved forward during the 1990s, climbing over barriers of culture and financial constraints to train hundreds of Kenyans and Americans and provide care in both urban hospital and rural clinic settings. All the while, the partners helped build the Moi University Faculty of Health Sciences (it would eventually change its name to Moi University School of Medicine) into a solid institution. But each year, a shadow was lengthening over Kenya and the rest of the African continent.

In the United States, the reported history of HIV/AIDS began in 1981 with a small notice in a Centers for Disease Control bulletin. The notice stated that a cluster of homosexual men in Los Angeles and New York had been diagnosed with Kaposi's sarcoma, a rare skin cancer, and pneumocystis carinii pneumonia, known as PCP. Soon, hundreds of gay men began dying in the United States of what was being called GRID (Gay-Related Immune Deficiency). By 1982, the disease was linked to blood and discovered to be also affecting heterosexual intravenous drug users, hemophiliacs, and recent immigrants from Haiti.

French researchers found the virus in 1983, and named it the human immunodeficiency virus, HIV. By 1985, the U.S. public began learning more about AIDS when thirteen-year-old HIV-positive hemophiliac Ryan White was barred from attending middle school in Kokomo, Indiana. That same year, actor Rock Hudson publicly acknowledged his AIDS diagnosis and died soon afterwards, making him one of over five thousand Americans to die of the disease in 1985 alone.

It was not known at the time, but these U.S. incidents were not HIV's debut. Later analysis of a blood sample of a man who had died in the Belgian Congo in 1959 showed the earliest confirmed case of HIV infection. Genomic records now reveal that the virus existed in humans in Africa as far back as the 1920s, when it was transferred from a chimpanzee, likely during butchering. Cases of "slim" had been observed in communities along the shores of Lake Victoria in Uganda, Tanzania, and Rwanda since the late 1970s. But the disease later recognized to be HIV/AIDS did not begin to spread significantly throughout Africa until the mid 1980s. In 1986, Rwanda conducted the first African national survey of HIV prevalence, and found that nearly one in five adults in the country's urban areas were HIV-positive. By 1990, an estimated five million Africans were infected with HIV.

HIV is a retrovirus, meaning it has a single-stranded RNA (ribonucleic acid) genome rather than the typical two-stranded loop of DNA (deoxyribonucleic acid). The virus is spread from one person to another through the transfer of blood, semen, vaginal fluid, pre-ejaculate, or breast milk. Once the virus enters the body, it attaches to and then ingratiates itself into white blood cells called lymphocytes, or CD4+ T cells, which play a crucial role in the body's immune system. Once it has found a way into the cell, HIV begins making copies of itself, producing as many as 10,000 new viruses in each cell.

A newly infected person often experiences fever, fatigue, and other flu-like symptoms. But after a month or two, the body produces antibodies to the virus and the infected person becomes asymptomatic for as long as ten years or more. Eventually, though, the body can no longer make more CD4 cells to replace the ones damaged by HIV, and the virus begins breaking down immune systems. Opportunistic infections the body would normally be able to resist, like Kaposi's sarcoma, PCP, or tuberculosis, begin to emerge. When these opportunistic infections occur, or when the number of CD4 cells in a small drop of a patient's blood falls below 200 (a healthy person will have over 700 CD4 cells in that same-size drop of blood), the patient is considered to have AIDS.

None of this virology explains why one area of the world has been so disproportionately affected by HIV. Even though less than 10 percent of the world's population lives in sub-Saharan Africa, two-thirds of the world's HIV cases occur there. Since the beginning of the pandemic, more than 25 million Africans have died of AIDS, a number significantly larger than the entire population of Texas. In some southern African countries, among them Swaziland and Botswana, more than one of every three adults is HIV-positive.

One reason that AIDS has been such a scourge in Africa is that the virus has its most devastating effect on the poor, and Africa has far more than its share of global poverty. Africa is a diverse mix of fifty-three countries, some of which are performing better than others economically, but half of all Africans live on less than $1 per day. One in six African children die before age five, and a third of the continent's population is malnourished. Africa is home to women who face starvation for themselves and their children if they refuse philandering husbands, fatalistic men who have had little or no access to education about disease, and girls who are forced to sell sex in order to support themselves or their families. All of these desperate scenarios are disproportionately present in Africa, as is the resulting risk of AIDS.

The causes for this poverty are several. The practices of nineteenth- and twentieth-century colonialism, especially the disempowerment of Africans and the exacerbation of ethnic rivalries, continue to have a devastating ripple effect throughout the continent. The postcolonial era of independence in the mid–twentieth century ushered in new indigenous leadership, but the new leaders too often followed the same exploitative practices as their colonial predecessors. During the Cold War, the United States and the Soviet Union used Africa as a proxy for their struggle. The United States allowed dictators and kleptocrats like Mobutu Sese Seko of Zaire to strip their countries of resources, all the while enjoying U.S. support in return for their renunciation of communism. The Soviet Union responded in kind, backing leaders like Ethiopia's brutal Mengistu Haile Mariam after he overthrew the U.S.-supported Haile Selassie, who for his part had ignored the famine that killed hundreds of thousands of his citizens.

After the Cold War, brutal ethnic violence continued in many African countries, hand in hand with political leadership that was inefficient at best and corrupt at worst. Even after the international community began to focus its efforts in Africa on reducing poverty, many of those efforts only exacerbated the problems. Burdened with billions of dollars of debt to the International Monetary Fund and the World Bank, many African countries were forced by these agencies to engage in "structural adjustment" policies to privatize and deregulate their economies. But the resulting loss of public-sector jobs and imposition of unaffordable user fees for health services had devastating effects on the poorest of the poor.

Kenya's first postcolonial leader was Jomo Kenyatta, who was elected president in late 1963; Kenyatta had helped lead the resistance against white settlers that effectively convinced the British government to hand over power to a democratically elected African government. Kenyatta, who held office until his death in 1978, led the new country to relative prosperity even as he routinely showed favoritism to members of his Kikuyu ethnic group and responded quickly and severely to dissenting voices. Kenyatta was succeeded by his vice president, Daniel arap Moi, a former schoolteacher who belonged to the Kalenjin ethnic group. During Moi's twenty-four years in power, Kenya continued to enjoy relative political stability, compared to many other African nations. But Moi maintained his primacy in part by jailing political opponents and suppressing dissent, all while amassing a personal fortune. By the time Moi left office in 2002, he had used his position to gather enough property and business interests to be widely considered one of the wealthiest men in Africa.

Moi's voluntary relinquishment of power in 2002 was a landmark event for Kenya's government, but his departure and the election of Mwai Kibaki did not solve all of Kenya's governance problems. Official corruption continued to plague the country, and in 2006, the Kibaki government admitted it had ordered a raid by masked gunmen that briefly shut down *The Standard* newspaper and the Kenya Television Network, which had been critical of the president. A 2007 editorial in the *Daily Nation*, Kenya's largest newspaper, commented on the state of Kenyan political leadership: "We admire those who can acquire the most in the shortest period of time—in our case, five years in Parliament, it seems, is the fastest track to instant wealth . . . Our leaders neither inspire us, nor the rest of the world. This is because we have made greed rather than responsibility the motivating force that drives our society."

In Kenya and throughout Africa, the toxic mix of colonialism, ethnic rivalries, and corruption meant that precious little government money was available for HIV prevention, education, or treatment when the AIDS pandemic was gathering steam in the 1990s. The governance problems hurt the prospects for donations, too, as many potential suppliers of aid were turned off by the prospect of their dollars being appropriated by corrupt government officials.

Even when some money was available for HIV intervention, progress was impeded by cultural barriers. In many areas of Africa, patriarchal ethnic customs gave free rein to the sexual appetites of men, while according their wives no ability to negotiate safe-sex practices. Religious influences, including the teachings of the Roman Catholic Church, discouraged condom use. And even though studies have shown that Africans on average are no more sexually active than Americans or Europeans, nor do they have more lifetime sex partners, the common African practice of keeping those partners concurrently helped spread HIV.

Dr. Mabel Nangami, a professor at Moi University's School of Public Health who earned her Ph.D. in sociology from the University of North Carolina, points to the African practice of polygamy as an example of cultural traditions mixing with modern economic burdens to create an ideal breeding ground for HIV. "With the westernization or modernization of Africa, direct polygamy is less common than it once was," Nangami said. "But instead of a man having three or four wives, he is often just taking that many mistresses. Boys are still taught to be sexually aggressive, and we still have this notion that you are not a man unless you can demonstrate that you can keep three women."

Nangami says that public education efforts encouraging "zero grazing"—the middle "B" in the iconic "ABC" campaigns urging HIV prevention through Abstinence, Be Faithful, and Condoms—are blunted by the forced separation many African married couples endure. "This western part of Kenya is extremely poor, and also extremely reliant on agriculture, maize in particular. When prices go down or adverse weather comes through, it may force the husband to move to urban areas to find work." When the man settles in Nairobi or another city, or if he takes work as a long-distance truck driver, he often finds other sexual partners—sometimes young girls who have also fled the hungry countryside and end up as commercial sex workers. But the husband still returns routinely to his wife and family, often taking the virus home with him.

For example, Rose Birgen's husband left their home in the rural Nandi district of western Kenya in the late 1990s to find work as a police officer at the international airport in Mombasa, on the country's Indian Ocean coast. Birgen stayed home with their children while her husband was away for weeks and months at a time. Twice she traveled to Mombasa and found him with another woman. Birgen's husband soon became sick with an illness he refused to discuss with his wife. After he died, Birgen was tested and learned she was HIV-positive. This concurrent-sexual-partner phenomenon is even more common in southern Africa, where men go to work in mines for months and years on end—and where the prevalence of HIV is the highest in the world.

"The wife at home is called the 'grass-cutter,'" Nangami says. "She is the one who not only takes care of the mother-in-law, but she symbolically and literally cuts the grass around the doorstep so the snakes won't bite when the man returns home." Cultural norms in most Kenyan societies require women to submit to patently unequal sexual arrangements. "You have to give your husband sex anytime he wants, even if you think he has been sleeping with others," Nangami says. She recalls her own pre-wedding conversation with her grandmother, who insisted that Nangami's university degree and postgraduate studies did not relieve her of this traditional obligation. "She told me that I had to submit to my husband no matter what I was doing, even if I was cooking or sewing or whatever."

Nangami laughs now at her grandmother's edict, but says that defiance of ethnic norms, such as the practice of a man "inheriting" his recently widowed sister-in-law, is no laughing matter. In the Luhya ethnic group, Nangami points out, failure to comply with such norms can cause a woman and her family to be treated as outcasts in their own village.

Nangami's critique of ethnic cultures' role in spreading HIV is accompanied by harsh words for the influence of western Christian churches, especially the prevalent Roman Catholic and Seventh-day Adventist congregations. "For a long time, the churches in Kenya did not accept the reality of HIV/AIDS, and instead told people they would be fine if they just stayed in the church. The church leaders blocked sex education, because they believed it encouraged promiscuity. And they preached Bible passages that commanded women to be submissive. All of this added to the stigma, and many people in the church who had HIV did not disclose it, which fueled the spread of the virus." Nangami points out that as recently as 2006, Kenyan first lady Lucy Kibaki, who like her husband, President Mwai Kibaki, is a Roman Catholic, told schoolgirls in Nairobi that she opposed the use of condoms. In 2007, the Catholic archbishop of nearby Mozambique told the BBC he believed some European-made condoms, and even antiretroviral drugs, are deliberately infected with HIV.

✿

By the late 1990s, no one living in Eldoret, much less practicing medicine there, could ignore the increasing death toll. "We were all aware of the AIDS crisis, but like so many others we saw it as such an overwhelming problem, we didn't know what we could do about it," Einterz said, "Some of us had the same defeatist attitudes we ended up fighting against later." But after it became clear in late 2000 that Daniel Ochieng was going to fully recover, whatever defeatist attitudes remained among Indiana and Moi physicians began to be replaced by horror and regret over the fate of patients like Akiru.

Akiru was a twenty-three-year-old woman who, just a few months after Daniel Ochieng's release from Moi Teaching and Referral Hospital, traveled to the Eldoret hospital all the way from Turkana in northern Kenya. With her was her three-year-old daughter, Ekipetot. By the time she made it to the hospital, Akiru's body was already wasted with tuberculosis and HIV. She had no money for even an HIV test, so Joe Mamlin paid out of his pocket for the tests that confirmed the obvious diagnosis. Although Mamlin could do little for her, Akiru stayed on the ward with her daughter, who lived at the foot of her mother's cot. As the days and weeks went by and Akiru grew sicker, everyone in the hospital became attached to her child. Mamlin regularly brought little Ekipetot to a small shop near the hospital to get a *mandazi,* a doughnut-like treat.

One morning when Mamlin was doing rounds in the hospital, he approached Akiru's bed, only to see that she had just died. He saw Ekipetot on the bed, too; still smiling while holding and tugging at her mother's hand. The veteran of forty-plus years of medicine could not hold back his tears. "I find this to be the most difficult task of my entire career," Mamlin wrote back to Indiana. "Every person of conscience would feel outrage if they could see what I'm seeing every day."

Einterz agreed. "We all need to be doing more: the U.S. government, institutions, all of us," he told a newspaper reporter in 2001. "I'm afraid we are going to look back on our time 200 years from now and say that this epidemic raged on, we could have stopped it, yet we chose to stand by and let it happen."

But in sub-Saharan Africa in 2001, there were a million good reasons not to start an HIV treatment program, most of them beginning with dollar signs. A month's worth of antiretroviral treatment cost 60,000 Kenyan shillings, then the equivalent of about $1,000. That amount was twice as much as a Kenyan doctor's monthly salary and twenty times a Kenyan farmer's monthly wages.

Mamlin's e-mails home, however, continued to close with the Reinhold Niebuhr quote invoking hope for the future. Mamlin describes himself as an "armchair theologian and philosopher" and often jokes that he is still trying to overcome his Southern Baptist roots. While in Kenya, Mamlin reread Paul Tillich's three-volume *Systematic Theology* cover to cover twice, along with generous helpings of Kierkegaard and Niebuhr. Amidst the death and desperation of a country caught up in the world's worst pandemic, Mamlin found some promise in those pages. "Most people only see the future as some construct of past events," he says. "They can't imagine the possibilities of change. But I always try to make myself vulnerable to new ideas."

Mamlin's friends and colleagues repeatedly refer to his ability to look past the horizon and envision future developments. His childhood friend Jim Greene explains the trait in the context of Stephen Covey's book on time management and prioritizing, *First Things First*. "Covey points out that most people concentrate their efforts on what is urgent and important, but truly transformative work is done in another area—efforts that are not urgent but important. Joe embodies the ability to cover both. It would have been easy for him to just treat any HIV-positive patient he could afford to care for, but he also focused on building a structure that would treat a whole region of people." Greene, a medical anthropologist who teaches at Wilkes Community College in West Jefferson, North Carolina, says that he has observed few physicians with this quality. "They tend to be focused on the individual patient, which is entirely appropriate, but Joe has always been broader than that."

As Mamlin contemplated the challenge of treating HIV/AIDS in Kenya, he was able to draw upon his experience building a citywide clinical care system and university medical group in Indianapolis. "I'm not scared of big numbers," he says. "At Wishard Hospital, we went from no outreach at all to twenty-one sites. We went from just me [in the Indiana University Medical Group] to one hundred physicians. I've learned that vision attracts funding. If it is the right idea at the right time, the funding will follow.

"Here in Kenya, in an environment where there are so many great needs and so few resources, I follow the lessons I learned in Indianapolis and Afghanistan."

So, in early 2001, Mamlin set up a small room in the Moi Teaching and Referral Hospital and began seeing HIV-positive patients, while he and Einterz wrote grants and begged individuals for money to buy the drugs the patients needed. As they made their pitches, the physicians gave the effort an ambitious-sounding name, the Academic Model for Prevention and Treatment of HIV/AIDS, or AMPATH. Some of the first patients in Mamlin's fledgling clinic were referred by Dr. Sylvester Kimaiyo, a Moi University professor who was leaving Eldoret for a year-long Merck fellowship in clinical pharmacology at Indiana University.

Kimaiyo grew up in the Nandi district, then still known as the "White Highlands," since black African ownership of the fertile land was illegal until Kenya's independence in 1963. Kimaiyo's family moved to Hoy's Bridge (later renamed Moi's Bridge by President Daniel arap Moi) when Kimaiyo, the eldest of ten children, began primary school. Kimaiyo's father was a mason whose schooling had stopped in fifth grade, and his mother was barely literate, but they were determined that their children be well-educated. Kimaiyo's siblings include a teacher, a pharmacist, and an informatics specialist. Another brother, who like Kimaiyo and their father before them stands well over six feet tall, was on the Kenyan national basketball and track teams.

Kimaiyo's own academic success began when his parents sent him to Lodwar Secondary School in the northern Kenya region of Turkana. Kimaiyo remembers traveling for two days on top of a large truck to reach Turkana, with the temperature rising as the truck slowly descended from his homeland's high altitude. "Secondary school was hot and hard and I missed my family," he says. "I had nothing to do but dedicate myself to my studies." His efforts earned him top marks, and his classmates took to calling Kimaiyo, who wore glasses from a young age, "the professor."

(Then and now, Kimaiyo's Kenyan colleagues chuckle at the incongruity of the given name for the studious physician. In the Nandi language, "Kimaiyo" is the word for alcohol, which is what his grandmother was brewing a batch of when his mother went into labor.)

Kimaiyo earned the Lodwar School's highest-ever mark on the Form 4 math/biology/chemistry exam, and he was selected for a spot at the prestigious St. Patrick's High School in Iten, operated by the Patrician Brothers of Ireland. After he earned the country's fifth-best score in the Kenyan Certificate of Secondary Education exam while at St. Patrick's, Kimaiyo enrolled in the medical school at the University of Nairobi.

Predictably, Kimaiyo excelled in his medical studies. After a fellowship at the London School of Tropical Medicine, where he studied the connections between HIV/AIDS and tuberculosis, he returned to western Kenya to teach and practice medicine as a member of the Moi University faculty. Kimaiyo, whose gentle manner and disarming smile softens the impression of his powerful intellect, soon earned a reputation among colleagues and students as one of the top medical teachers in all of Kenya.

But when Kimaiyo's younger sister Roselyn fell ill while working in Nairobi in the late 1990s, even Kenya's rising medical star could not save her. Roselyn, a banker and former track and basketball star, wasted away before his eyes. "She was diagnosed with cryptococcal meningitis, and we could treat her for that," Kimaiyo said. "But it was clear she had AIDS, even though no one talked about it. It was 1998, and there were no drugs to be had. So I went and got her and brought her back to an Eldoret hospital, where we took care of her for two months." In 1997, Roselyn died at the age of thirty-one.

As he saw more patients with AIDS on the Moi Teaching and Referral Hospital wards, Kimaiyo's grief mixed with frustration. Over two-thirds of the hospital's beds were filled with patients, two or three lying head-to-foot in each bed, suffering from AIDS-related illnesses. "There really was no treatment for HIV patients then," Kimaiyo says. "Whenever we diagnosed HIV, we said, 'This is the end, it's HIV. Take them home to die, or have them stay in the wards to die.' And then we would move on to the next patient. It was just diagnosis and then almost literally signing the death certificate."

When Kimaiyo left for his year-long fellowship in the United States, he transferred any HIV patients he could to Mamlin's new clinic. But even after settling in at Indiana, Kimaiyo was unable to shake the images of his generation of Kenyans lying in huts and hospital beds, wasting away from HIV/AIDS.

During that year in Indianapolis, Kimaiyo discussed AIDS with a U.S. newspaper reporter. "There is an incredibly high stigma that our culture attaches to having HIV," he said, explaining that the disease marked a person as promiscuous and unclean. "Very few people will admit to having the disease. If I make the diagnosis with the husband, even educated men will try to keep me from telling their wives. Some men have been infected for years and never tell their wives. At funerals for people who died of AIDS, they go to great lengths to blame another disease." Kimaiyo also echoed Mabel Nangami's criticism of the patriarchal nature of Kenyan society, which tolerates a high level of male promiscuity and also objects to condom use for cultural and religious reasons.

But Kimaiyo insisted to the newspaper reporter that culture was not solely to blame for the pandemic. At least equally responsible, he said, was the country's grinding poverty, which forced young girls—often AIDS orphans themselves—into prostitution, where they often contracted and spread the disease. Poverty was also leaving Kenyans without access to HIV treatment readily available in western countries. Kimaiyo said that the inability to afford treatment fueled the spread of AIDS, since most of his patients saw little point in being tested for a disease they could never afford to get treated. "If I want to test a patient who has symptoms that make me suspect HIV, many will tell me, 'If you know I am HIV-positive, you can't treat me anyway,'" Kimaiyo said. "So they would rather not go through the psychological trauma of knowing. They leave, and they won't come back until they have full-blown AIDS. By then, they have spread the disease."

Kimaiyo did not have a license to practice medicine in the United States during his fellowship, so he began spending most of his time in the Indiana University School of Medicine laboratories. Although his fellowship called for him to study cardiology drugs, his attention kept drifting to the antiretroviral medicines used to treat HIV. Kimaiyo learned what drugs Mamlin was prescribing for his HIV patients in Kenya, got a key to the lab, and would sometimes spend all night studying the drugs. He began attending an Indianapolis HIV treatment clinic with physician Joe Wheat, the infectious disease specialist at the Indiana University School of Medicine who guided and supported Mamlin's treatment of Daniel Ochieng. Soon, Kimaiyo had had clinical and laboratory exposure to HIV treatment that almost no other African physician had been able to obtain. By the time he returned to Kenya in 2002, Kimaiyo had put aside his cardiology plans. Instead, he joined Mamlin in the HIV clinic at Moi Hospital and then opened his own AMPATH clinic, becoming one of the first African physicians to routinely provide treatment for HIV/AIDS.

❋

In the summer of 2002, just a few months after Kimaiyo set up the second AMPATH clinic, the Indiana and Moi physicians finally won their first big grant award. The MTCT-Plus Initiative (MTCT stands for Mother-to-Child-Transmission of HIV/AIDS), a program sponsored by a coalition of foundations, awarded the Indiana–Moi program one of just twelve international grants given in the developing world. The grant provided for HIV care and treatment for mothers, children, and other family members, and included a commitment to lifetime treatment of enrolled patients. The Indiana–Moi team used the grant and other private donations to begin enrolling more HIV-positive patients, with the goal of treating 1,000 Kenyans for life.

By the time of these first Indiana–Moi tentative steps toward funding treatment of HIV/AIDS, global AIDS activists, world governments, and funders had already spent several years engaged in a grim debate about priorities. The question was whether it was more important to focus on preventing HIV in the developing world or to treat the millions otherwise destined to die from the disease. But the Indiana–Moi doctors refused to accept an either/or position in the debate, insisting that treatment and prevention are natural partners.

Their case in point was AMPATH Patient #1, Daniel Ochieng, who by now was working as the leader of an AMPATH effort to reach out to the HIV-infected Kenyan population. Ochieng and many other Kenyans agreed with Kimaiyo that HIV/AIDS stigma, which blocked widespread testing and safe-sex practices, was less of a cultural phenomenon than a predictable reaction to the prevailing African view that the disease was the equivalent of a death sentence. In other words, treatment *is* prevention. "Knowing there is treatment for the disease makes people take the test," Ochieng said.

So Ochieng and colleagues like Rose Birgen, the HIV survivor who had lost her husband and later an infant child to the disease, led community meetings to advocate condom use, responsible sexual practices, and testing. At those meetings, the speakers' most compelling argument was their own obvious good health. "We show ourselves to the community that we are HIV-positive yet we are living, and we reduce the stigma," Birgen said. "When we go to *baraza*s [community meetings] today, they go to be tested tomorrow."

By early 2003, more than 80 percent of new mothers treated at the Moi Hospital were agreeing to be tested for HIV, and Indiana–Moi surveys showed that many of the culture's deadly HIV myths were fading away. Over three-quarters of Kenyans surveyed knew that someone without symptoms can transmit HIV, and almost all knew there was no cure for the disease. Less than 5 percent bought into the dangerous fallacies that HIV has a supernatural cause or can be cured by sex with a virgin.

As the Indiana–Moi program's treatment numbers started to climb, global health experts took notice. "There is a growing sense that devoting a lot of resources to treatment is necessary, but there is not a lot out there yet in how to do it responsibly," Dr. Tim Evans, director of health equity for the Rockefeller Foundation, told an Indianapolis newspaper in 2003. "That is why the IU–Moi model is so important. It is the best practice model, which importantly is not a Cadillac that no one can afford. It is a Toyota that is a good quality model of care that can be replicated in a lot of settings with constrained resources."

Evans and others were concerned about the uniquely thorny challenge presented by treating HIV in the developing world. Even if the price of antiretroviral drugs dropped all the way to zero, this was not the kind of emergency relief that could be handed out like sacks of rice from the back of a United Nations truck. HIV-positive patients have to be educated and supported in their drug-taking regimen, and there has to be a lifetime supply. Poor compliance with the regimen can lead to a strain of HIV that is resistant to the triple-drug cocktail and responsive only to prohibitively expensive alternative drug combinations. As bad as the HIV/AIDS situation in sub-Saharan Africa was, sloppy treatment efforts could make it even worse.

Fear of this potentially catastrophic result was as significant a barrier as lack of funds in keeping lifesaving drugs out of the developing world. So if the pandemic was to be halted, there first needed to be a protocol for effective and affordable HIV care in countries that have precious little in the way of traditional health resources. When the Indiana–Moi team started treating patients who wrapped their space-age medication in scarves and carried them down muddy red paths to thatch-roofed huts, the physicians were quite self-consciously creating a model for treatment that could be applied to the entire developing world.

"This is a program that is reversing the tide of skepticism regarding providing treatment," Evans said in 2003. "Their success is very, very timely. The people working on this program are public health heroes. They are doing things that many people thought could never be done, and it is going to have a huge multiplier effect."

Evans was to offer much more to AMPATH than words of praise. When visiting Eldoret in late 2002, Evans learned from Mamlin and Kimaiyo that the budding model was facing a cash crisis. "Our original pilot funding was winding down and we had dozens of patients hanging on with no antiretroviral therapy," Mamlin says. When Evans told the newspaper about the "multiplier effect" of AMPATH's success, he was echoing the increasing talk about a large-scale global commitment to HIV treatment in sub-Saharan Africa. Einterz, Mamlin, and Kimaiyo had heard the talk, too. But while they waited and hoped for the big news to come, they were running out of money and medicine, and facing the prospect of losing momentum and morale—not to mention the lives of their at-risk patients.

Evans suggested that AMPATH write a proposal to the Purpleville Foundation, a small family foundation in Canada. Neither Einterz nor Mamlin had ever heard of it, but they gave it a try. Referring to the talk of generous grant funding for HIV care that seemed to be on the horizon, they wrote, "AMPATH will eventually realize its goals. But the number of young people and children lost during this gap of time between our pilot phase and access to funding for scale-up will needlessly add to the absurd tragedy now gripping East Africa."

Large-scale government support was indeed forthcoming, and would form the core of AMPATH's move from caring for just Daniel Ochieng in 2001 to serving 70,000 HIV-positive patients by the end of 2008. But it was smaller private donors that funded Indiana University's initial foray into Kenya and the first efforts to train patients with job skills and improved agricultural practices. It was individual gifts that built an operating room for Moi Hospital and AMPATH's first rural clinic. And it was the previously unknown Purpleville Foundation that in early 2003 gave $500,000 to AMPATH in response to the grant request, which was titled "A Bridge of Hope."

"They have a special place in the hearts of all connected with AMPATH," Mamlin says. "I find it hard to say how we got from here to there without Purpleville in the equation."

"SELDOM HAS HISTORY OFFERED A GREATER OPPORTUNITY"

ON JUNE 7, 2001, REPRESENTATIVE Henry Hyde, then the chair of the International Relations Committee of the U.S. House of Representatives, convened a hearing to discuss his new global AIDS bill, which included a pilot program for purchasing and delivering antiretroviral drugs. But the hearing on the Global Access to HIV/AIDS Prevention, Awareness, Education and Treatment Act started on a sour note with the testimony of Andrew Natsios, recently confirmed as President George W. Bush's administrator for the U.S. Agency for International Development (USAID), and a veteran of USAID from the George H. W. Bush administration. Natsios told the committee that the United States was better off focusing on the prevention aspects of global AIDS, since treatment of the 25 million people infected with HIV in sub-Saharan Africa was virtually impossible:

> People [in Africa] do not know what watches and clocks are. They do not use Western means for telling time. They use the sun. These drugs have to be administered during a certain se-

quence of time during the day. And when you say, "take it at ten o'clock," people will say "what do you mean ten o'clock?" They don't use those terms in the villages to describe time. They describe morning and afternoon and evening. So that's a problem.

Natsios's testimony stoked immediate controversy. Advocates pointed out that he was wrong in several of his stated premises for pessimism about treatment, which included a supposition that the antiretroviral medicine needed to be frozen and that there are no roads in Africa. Several African advocacy groups and members of the Congressional Black Caucus called for Natsios to resign. In his excellent book, *The Invisible People: How the U.S. Slept through the Global AIDS Pandemic, the Greatest Humanitarian Catastrophe of Our Time,* Greg Behrman reports that United Nations secretary-general Kofi Annan intentionally arrived forty-five minutes late for a subsequent meeting with Natsios. "I'm sorry," the Nobel laureate from Ghana said with undisguised sarcasm. "I've been having trouble telling time."

But however clumsy he was in stating his rationale, Natsios's gloomy view of the possibility of treatment accurately reflected much of the conventional—and fatalistic—wisdom about how the international community and the United States should approach the HIV/AIDS pandemic. Two months before Natsios's testimony, the *Washington Post* quoted an unnamed global health official reflecting on the crisis and saying, "It's so politically incorrect to say, but we may have to sit by and just see these millions of [HIV-infected] people die." Even a year after Natsios's testimony, the prestigious British medical journal *Lancet* published an article by AIDS researchers saying that any new funding to address the HIV/AIDS crisis must be allocated to prevention efforts instead of antiretroviral treatment for those already infected.

The reluctance to support treatment had bipartisan roots, as global AIDS had not been a priority for the Clinton administration either. "It is hard to explain that moral failing [during the Clinton presidency]," Allen Moore, formerly the legislative director for Senator Bill Frist and now a senior fellow at the Global Health Council, said in a 2007 address to the Johns Hopkins Bloomberg School of Public Health. "Some of it was ignorance; some was indifference; some was politics. There was no call to action by the President nor was there any bi-partisan political consensus to move forward aggressively."

At the time of Natsios's testimony in mid-2001, the second President Bush seemed no more willing than Clinton to pursue a course that would include AIDS treatment in sub-Saharan Africa. "I don't know [Natsios] very well personally," says Dr. Joe O'Neill, who would become director of Bush's Office of National AIDS Policy a year after the testimony. "But his statement reflected his agency. USAID was just not interested in HIV treatment."

Remarkably, it was just nineteen months later, in the State of the Union address he delivered at the U.S. Capitol on January 28, 2003, that Natsios's boss, President Bush, dramatically announced the largest commitment ever by one nation toward a single international disease—and HIV treatment was the very core of Bush's historic pledge:

> Today, on the continent of Africa, nearly 30 million people have the AIDS virus—including 3 million children under the age 15. There are whole countries in Africa where more than one-third of the adult population carries the infection. More than 4 million require immediate drug treatment. Yet across that continent, only 50,000 AIDS victims—only 50,000—are receiving the medicine they need.
>
> Because the AIDS diagnosis is considered a death sentence, many do not seek treatment. Almost all who do are turned away. A doctor in rural South Africa describes his frustration. He says, "We have no medicines. Many hospitals tell people, you've got AIDS, we can't help you. Go home and die." In an age of miraculous medicines, no person should have to hear those words.
>
> AIDS can be prevented. Anti-retroviral drugs can extend life for many years. And the cost of those drugs has dropped from $12,000 a year to under $300 a year—which places a tremendous possibility within our grasp. Ladies and gentlemen, seldom has history offered a greater opportunity to do so much for so many.
>
> We have confronted, and will continue to confront, HIV/ AIDS in our own country. And to meet a severe and urgent crisis abroad, tonight I propose the Emergency Plan for AIDS Relief—a work of mercy beyond all current international ef-

forts to help the people of Africa. This comprehensive plan will prevent 7 million new AIDS infections, treat at least 2 million people with life-extending drugs, and provide humane care for millions of people suffering from AIDS, and for children orphaned by AIDS.

I ask the Congress to commit $15 billion over the next five years, including nearly $10 billion in new money, to turn the tide against AIDS in the most afflicted nations of Africa and the Caribbean.

This nation can lead the world in sparing innocent people from a plague of nature.

The portion of Bush's speech dedicated to AIDS was interrupted by bipartisan congressional applause several times, and the images on television included the first lady standing with Dr. Peter Mugyenyi, who directs an HIV clinic in Uganda. Just four months later, the President's Emergency Plan for AIDS Relief (by then commonly referred to by the acronym PEPFAR) won congressional approval and was quickly signed into law. As of the end of 2007, the United States had provided the lifesaving antiretroviral treatment once thought impossible to over one million people in fifteen countries in sub-Saharan Africa, Asia, and the Caribbean. PEPFAR has reached millions more with intervention to prevent mother-to-child transmission of HIV.

The groundwork for the State of the Union PEPFAR announcement had been laid very quietly within the Bush administration. Even the advocates who devoted their lives to the cause of AIDS treatment were stunned when the president announced the ambitious goals of the new program. "If anyone told you that they knew how big and bold it [PEPFAR] was going to be, they would be misleading you," says David Gartner, policy director for the Global AIDS Alliance, who had previously worked on global AIDS issues as a Senate staffer and with rock star Bono's DATA (Debt AIDS Trade Africa) organization. Gartner listened to the State of the Union address on the radio, and when he heard the breadth of Bush's commitment and the blunt statement to the world that HIV-infected persons should not be sent home to die, Gartner cried. "I was pretty overwhelmed," he says. "It took a lot to get there, and there was a lot still to go through, but that was a huge moment."

Huge indeed: This six-paragraph statement in the State of the Union address saved the lives of some of the sickest, poorest, and most geographically and geopolitically remote persons on earth, and may be seen some day as one of history's greatest human rights and global health triumphs. But it was also diametrically opposed to the Bush administration position delivered by Natsios to Congress less than two years before, and Gartner was far from alone in being stunned by the announcement. Only a few media accounts have covered the dramatic shift, and they attribute the birth of PEPFAR either to the ministrations of a rock star (Bono) or a mega-pastor (Franklin Graham), or to President Bush's desire to balance the "hard power" of the buildup to the Iraq War with the "soft power" of a sweeping humanitarian initiative. A closer look shows that, even taken together, these explanations for PEPFAR's creation are accurate yet incomplete.

※

In his speech, President Bush specifically noted the marked drop in the cost of antiretroviral (ARV) treatment. There is no question that the scale of PEPFAR, if not its very existence, would have been impossible if ARV therapy had remained as expensive and complicated as it was in the late 1990s. At that time, the most common drug regimen consisted of taking a half dozen or more pills at different times of the day at a cost of over $1,000 per month. This complex routine was apparently fresh in the mind of Andrew Natsios when he delivered his June 2001 congressional testimony. According to a colleague, Natsios and his wife had personally cared for a friend suffering from AIDS several years before. During his infamous testimony, Natsios was apparently generalizing from that very vivid experience to the challenges facing the African continent.

At the turn of the twenty-first century, the treatment barriers of cost and complexity began to fall. Brazil and Argentina started providing generic AIDS drugs to their citizens at a fraction of the cost charged by patent-holding pharmaceutical companies. In 1998, South Africa began a process that would also have led to importing generic ARVs. Initially, a consortium of pharmaceutical companies sued to stop the South African government from bringing in the generics. But pressure from activists, the United Nations, and individual governments triggered concessions by the pharmaceutical companies, and they dismissed their lawsuit in 2001. The price of ARVs quickly dropped by 90 percent. At the same time, drug companies, in particular those that manufactured the generic versions, were able to combine several pills into one, greatly simplifying the treatment regimen. Suddenly, the dream of widespread HIV treatment seemed possible.

Some of the pressure to lower ARV prices was generated at high-profile international AIDS gatherings. At the 2000 International AIDS Conference in Durban, South Africa, former South African president Nelson Mandela defined the AIDS fight in moral terms, saying, "In this inter-dependent and globalized world, we have indeed again become the keepers of our brother and sister." Economist Jeffrey Sachs put a price tag on that obligation, a $10 billion per year global commitment of which the U.S. share would be $3 billion annually. Sachs's numbers seemed pie-in-the-sky at the time; he recounts that in early 2001, after presenting his case for $3 billion per year to Condoleezza Rice, then national security adviser, Bush's economic adviser Lawrence Lindsey congenially advised him, "Don't hold your breath."

Then, in June 2001, the very same month that Andrew Natsios made his gloomy prognostication for the chances of AIDS treatment in Africa, the United Nations convened a special session of the General Assembly on the topic of HIV/AIDS. It was the first time the body had ever been called together solely to address a specific health threat. The General Assembly, inspired by poignant pleas from African leaders, adopted a unanimous commitment of support for Kofi Annan's recently announced Global Fund to Fight HIV/AIDS, Malaria, and Tuberculosis. The following year, the World Health Organization and other UN agencies committed themselves to the goal of providing antiretroviral therapy for three million people by the end of 2005. By this time, programs like AMPATH and the Harvard-affiliated Partners in Health were demonstrating that HIV treatment could indeed be accomplished in the poorest of countries.

There was a growing international movement to provide

HIV/AIDS treatment in sub-Saharan Africa, and its core U.S. support came from two very different groups. The first group was the existing AIDS activist community, which had been successful in raising awareness and demanding government action for the domestic crisis and was now turning its attention to the global pandemic. Warren W. "Buck" Buckingham, a gay American man who has been living with HIV since the early 1980s, had worked exclusively on U.S. HIV/AIDS issues for fifteen years; he spent much of that time speaking out about the disease and administering federal HIV/AIDS funding for the Clinton administration. In 1998, Buckingham traveled to South Africa to visit some of the regions where as many as one in four adults were infected with HIV. "I came back from South Africa changed, and I knew I would devote the rest of the time I had left to the global response to AIDS," says Buckingham, who is now PEPFAR country coordinator for Kenya. "I was one of many activists who graduated from our own regional interests to realizing we had the ability to impact the lives of those infected around the world."

When their efforts expanded from the U.S. crisis to global AIDS, Buckingham and other traditional AIDS activists found themselves joined by an unlikely ally: the Christian evangelical movement. "There is no question that one of the critical components to the birth of PEPFAR was that there was a set of new players in the AIDS conversation," Buckingham says. "We probably do not yet have enough distance from the late 1990s and early 2000s to fully appreciate the role of evangelical groups in sounding the call at the White House and on Capitol Hill that AIDS was a moral issue." Evangelical Christians are usually defined as those who believe it is their obligation to proselytize their faith in the Bible as the literal truth and that acceptance of Jesus Christ is the exclusive path to salvation. In the United States, evangelicals are considered a strong voting bloc for the Republican Party, and were specifically identified by such conservative Republican lawmakers as Representative Henry Hyde, Senator Bill Frist, Senator Mike DeWine, and Senator Rick Santorum as inspiration for their support for global AIDS funding.

Evangelicals also had significant access to policy makers within the Bush administration. An October 2003 *New York Times* article, "Evangelicals Sway White House on Human Rights Issues Abroad," concluded that white evangelicals had raised the profile of AIDS within what *Times* reporter Elisabeth Bumiller called "one of the most religious White Houses in American history." An unnamed administration official was quoted in Derek Hodel's 2004 report for the Ford Foundation, *At the Crossroads: A Study of Federal HIV/AIDS Advocacy,* as affirming evangelicals' clout on the AIDS issue in the Oval Office: "Evangelical Christians [were] very important in getting the issue on the radar screen with the president—that Jesus would want us to do this—they were very influential in the president's thinking."

The most influential of those evangelicals was Franklin Graham, son of the renowned Reverend Billy Graham and founder of the faith-based organization Samaritan's Purse, which operates AIDS programs internationally. Graham met regularly with Bush's chief political aide Karl Rove, and was instrumental in bringing about the extraordinary about-face on AIDS by Senator Jesse Helms. Helms had once memorably labeled foreign aid a "rathole," and said in 1995 that the government should spend less money on people with AIDS because their illness was the result of "deliberate, disgusting, revolting conduct." But by February 2002, while addressing a Samaritan's Purse conference, Helms delivered an old-fashioned confessional and vow of repentance. "I'm ashamed I've done so little," he told the delegates. "I will do better than I have done in the past, and I will work with you." The next month, Helms announced his support for a U.S. commitment of $500 million to prevent mother-to-child transmission of HIV.

In 2001 and 2002, Helms had plenty of congressional company in expressing support for a significant increase in U.S. spending on the global AIDS crisis. Representative Hyde and Senator Frist on the Republican side of the aisle, along with Representative Barbara Lee and Senator John Kerry, both Democrats, proposed ambitious initiatives. Hyde's global AIDS legislation, whose treatment component was the subject of Andrew Natsios's June 2001 criticism, passed the House of Representatives in December of that same year. On its passage, Hyde spoke from the floor of the House to defend the necessity of HIV treatment:

The novel bilateral treatment program that my bill authorizes is vitally important, for it gives hope to those already suffering from AIDS. By authorizing a pilot treatment program, we can work to extend the productive lives of those infected by the virus. This is not only the right thing to do, it has beneficial impact on treatment as well. Without some expectation of care, the poor have little reason to be tested for AIDS or to seek help. I am fully cognizant of the challenge posed by treatment programs in developing countries. However, it is my hope that successful treatment programs such as those carried out by the AIDS Healthcare Foundation will be replicated in developing countries. Madam Speaker, there simply is no option other than treatment if we are ever to stem the tide of this pandemic.

By May 2002, the *New York Times* was reporting that "an unlikely alliance" of conservative and liberal members of Congress was ratcheting up the pressure on President Bush to increase AIDS spending. Congressional leaders like Senator Frist and House minority leader Richard Gephardt had recently witnessed the African AIDS crisis firsthand. "I came away knowing and believing that [AIDS] is the moral issue of our time," Gephardt told the *Times*.

The *Times* article was also one of many to note the influence of rock star Bono. The lead singer for the band U2 had spent years relentlessly leveraging his celebrity into access to lawmakers like President Bush, U.S. Treasury Secretary Paul O'Neill, and Senator Helms, whom Bono had first met to discuss global AIDS in the summer of 2001. Bono's activism raised the profile of the global AIDS struggle through such media coverage as a March 2002 *Time* magazine cover story entitled "Can Bono Save the World?" In commemoration of World AIDS Day in December 2002, Bono recruited fellow celebrities like Ashley Judd, Chris Tucker, Lance Armstrong, and Warren Buffett to join him on a seven-day, seven-city "Heart of America" tour of the U.S. Midwest. One of the cities was Indianapolis, where Bono met with Indiana–Moi's Bob Einterz. The tour intentionally targeted the political constituency of Bush and the Republican Congress with a message about the urgency of increasing AIDS funding and debt relief for African countries.

※

By this point, just a month before the announcement of PEP-FAR, it was not clear to activists, congressional leaders, and the media whether all of this activity was having significant effect inside the White House. President Bush had not been completely silent about the global AIDS crisis: he had pledged $200 million to the Global Fund to Fight HIV/AIDS, Malaria, and Tuberculosis in 2001 and $500 million to the prevention of mother-to-child HIV transmission in June 2002. But the latter announcement in particular generated as many jeers as cheers, with activists and members of Congress pointing out that less than half of the announced $500 million was an investment of new money. "If we follow the course the White House has charted, in just a few years we will be dealing with millions more poor, hungry, desperate orphans whose mothers have died from AIDS," said Senator Richard Durbin of Illinois.

Unbeknownst to Durbin, most of his fellow members of Congress, and the activist community, Dr. Joe O'Neill was even then in the midst of helping the president chart a very different course toward widespread HIV/AIDS treatment. O'Neill, a physician, describes himself as a career civil servant, having started working for the U.S. Department of Health and Human Services in 1989 and eventually directing the Ryan White Comprehensive AIDS Resource Emergency (CARE) program for four years during the Clinton administration. When O'Neill was first approached in 2002 about taking the position of director of the Office of National AIDS Policy, informally known as the "AIDS czar," in the George W. Bush administration, he was skeptical. "Bill Clinton did very, very little about global AIDS while he was in the White House, so my impression of the AIDS czar job was that it was a position of being a flak catcher from the AIDS activist community," O'Neill says. But Josh Bolten, then the deputy White House chief of staff, persuaded O'Neill that Bush was truly committed to significant action against global AIDS. O'Neill was also impressed by the potential hinted at by the early Bush promise to contribute $200 million to the Global Fund in 2001, a commitment made before the fund actually existed.

O'Neill accepted the position, and his lingering doubts were erased during his initial meeting with his new boss. "My first conversation with the president was supposed to just be a photo opportunity," he says. "When you work at the White House, you want a photo on the wall to show interest groups that you have the connection to the top. I was told the meeting was going to last only three minutes, but it ended up being a forty-five-minute talk that focused on my experience as an AIDS physician. The president asked about the Lazarus effect, and whether, in my experience with my clinic patients, the AIDS drugs really do have that dramatic effect.

"The length of this talk pushed back his calendar a ton, which is a big deal in the Bush White House, where the calendar is set in five-minute increments. The two points I took home from that meeting were one, that he really cares about this issue, and two, he really wanted to do something about it."

O'Neill, who was later described by Bush as "the architect" of PEPFAR, is careful to list many others who helped craft the program. But he does believe that his own experience as a practicing AIDS physician helped shape the treatment focus of PEPFAR. On Friday mornings while he worked as AIDS czar, O'Neill saw patients in a Johns Hopkins clinic, then went to the White House in the afternoon. "I was able to take the stories of AIDS in inner-city Baltimore to brief the president in context of policy discussions, which really made a difference," he says. "One of the reasons that PEPFAR is so strong on treatment is because I was treating people myself.

"Remember that, at this time, virtually no one was doing treatment in Africa. During one of my early conversations with him, I said, 'Mr. President, I don't have a lot of data to back me up right now, but I don't think you can do effective prevention if you do not do treatment. The reason is that the people in the community need hope. Why would you get tested if there is no treatment? I was able to cite him anecdotes from my own clinical experience about an HIV-positive test turning people's lives around—the times when it inspired them not just to get treatment, but to quit drugs or alcohol and clean up their act."

O'Neill's Oval Office advocacy seemed to work. He recalls a

moment at a subsequent meeting where an aide brought up the necessity of prevention funding and Bush replied, "You can't do effective prevention if you don't have a treatment program along with it," then looked over at O'Neill and nodded.

O'Neill and others involved in planning PEPFAR list many administration supporters for launching the ambitious AIDS response, including Bolten; Scott Evertz, O'Neill's predecessor; Anthony Fauci, director of the National Institute of Allergy and Infectious Diseases; physician and NIH researcher Mark Dybul (who would by 2006 become the U.S global AIDS coordinator implementing PEPFAR); Deputy Secretary of State Dr. Jack Chow; White House domestic policy advisers Jay Lefkowitz and Margaret Spellings; National Security Council staffer Jendayi Frazer; and such cabinet-level players as Secretary of Health and Human Services Tommy Thompson and National Security Adviser Condoleezza Rice. Bush's chief speechwriter, Michael Gerson, a high-profile evangelical Christian who was close to the president, was also an advocate for PEPFAR. A *New Yorker* magazine profile of Gerson, and then Gerson's own book, *Heroic Conservatism*, noted that Gerson once told the president and other advisers gathered to discuss the pros and cons of an ambitious global AIDS effort, "If we can do this, and we don't, it will be a source of shame."

Early on, the administration's most eloquent public voice on global AIDS was Secretary of State Colin Powell. After a May 2001 trip to Africa, Powell told the UN General Assembly Special Session on HIV/AIDS, "I was a soldier, but I know of no enemy in war more insidious or vicious than AIDS, an enemy that poses a clear and present danger to the world."

Considerations of domestic and international politics helped move the Bush administration's global AIDS plans forward. Administration officials say that responding to the evangelical base of Bush voters and reaching out to African American voters were both key priorities for Karl Rove, who saw PEPFAR as pleasing both constituencies. As the scope and direction of PEPFAR was being debated, a January 2003 trip by Bush to Africa loomed, during which he would be expected to announce a significant commitment to the region. Although the Africa trip was ultimately postponed, the buildup to a U.S. invasion of Iraq, far and away the highest-profile international issue of the day, intersected with the PEPFAR plans. During the 2003 State of the Union address, after Bush announced PEPFAR, he immediately segued to outlining his plans for the U.S. role in combating international terrorism, including a lengthy recitation of the case for a preemptive war with Iraq. (That recitation included the infamously inaccurate assertion that Saddam Hussein had tried to buy uranium from Niger.) The speech's juxtaposition of breathtaking U.S. humanitarian outreach and the controversial aggression toward Iraq was clearly not accidental. "I was told by administration officials that PEPFAR's announcement in the State of the Union was very much a 'hard power/soft power' thing," says Sarah Jane Hise of the Center for Global Development, a leading think tank on international poverty policy.

But Joe O'Neill stresses that the obvious political considerations for PEPFAR's creation and timing should not overshadow the fact that the bold step on HIV/AIDS enjoyed wide support in the Bush administration. "I remember walking out of one meeting where this was all taking its final shape, and several of us had tears in our eyes," O'Neill says. "One of my colleagues said to us that this may be the most important thing we [the Bush administration] will ever do."

PEPFAR was not a difficult sell within the White House staff, O'Neill says, because Bush himself never wavered in his intent to make a significant dollar commitment. "The message I got from day one from the president was that global AIDS was a huge problem and that he did not want it to go unaddressed on his watch," O'Neill says. "The highest number [for U.S. global AIDS plans] I asked for was $15 billion, and that is what he committed to."

❧

Before the announcement of PEPFAR, only O'Neill and a handful of others in the Bush administration were aware of the breadth of the HIV/AIDS plans under consideration, and all were sworn to secrecy. In the months before the State of the Union address, O'Neill had to stonewall longtime AIDS administrators in other executive agencies, not to mention AIDS activists and congressional leaders, who were worried about the president's inaction. The lack of outside involvement in the planning stage has led to some suggestion that the Bush White House created PEPFAR without regard to activist or congressional pressure on the administration to respond more forcefully to the global AIDS crisis. An unnamed administration official told Derek Hodel for his *At the Crossroads* report, "The administration really wanted to listen, but activists made a mistake by being negative—because it felt so good to be negative, because they hate this president— they failed to identify when they did have common ground, and therefore lost their opportunity to participate. The traditional groups could have gotten involved had they been willing to be- come engaged on the substantive issue of global AIDS—but by insisting on making it political, they lost that opportunity."

Former Frist aide Allen Moore agrees that advocates did not influence PEPFAR's creation. "If the advocates were so effective, why did they have so little impact on President Clinton?" asks Moore. "In my judgment, the prime motivator for PEPFAR was facts on the ground, not advocacy. In sub-Saharan Africa and elsewhere, unprecedented death, devastation, and instability were made worse by the failure to do more in the 1990s. That is what set the table for something big—something like PEPFAR."

O'Neill echoes that analysis, even as he gives credit to the po- litical influence of evangelicals who elevated the profile of AIDS within the White House. "I'm a big fan of AIDS activism," says O'Neill, who is openly gay. "I was taking care of patients in San Francisco General in the 1980s, and I know we would not be where we are without AIDS activism. But the more vocal and aggressive AIDS activists had essentially no impact on this pro- gram."

Policy makers are historically and understandably reluctant to bestow credit on activists who have harangued them for years. But it is clear that the activism on global AIDS had a significant role in inspiring PEPFAR. For one thing, although there was a clear distinction between the advocates who were welcome in the Oval Office (evangelical preachers, rock stars, pioneering AIDS physicians, etc.) and those who were picketing at the gates of the White House, activists of both categories regularly combined forces. Bono's 2002 Heart of America tour was managed in part by advocates associated with the more aggressive Global AIDS Alliance, and the ambitious treatment figures supported by Franklin Graham and others in their White House lobbying were supplied by more socially liberal economists and advocates. "The push for a greater global AIDS response had the broadest base of advocacy groups—Christian conservatives, students, domestic HIV/AIDS groups—that I have ever seen on any development issue," says Sarah Jane Hise.

Those advocacy groups point out that the buildup to PEP-FAR included a carrot-and-stick approach to inspiring the Bush administration to action. The carrot of incentive came from the promise of domestic and international political gains earned through an ambitious global AIDS program, while ugly demonstrations and embarrassing publicity provided the stick of negative reinforcement for any perceived neglect of the suffering millions. In 2002 alone, global AIDS activists regularly picketed the White House, staged a demonstration in Senator John Kerry's office, held a large rally in Washington, stormed the stage during Secretary Thompson's address to the International AIDS Conference in Barcelona, and booed O'Neill when he addressed the U.S. Conference on AIDS.

As the Bush administration began to make some commitments to global AIDS through its pledges to the Global Fund and to preventing mother-to-child transmission, the activist community responded not with gratitude but with an insistence that the bar remain much higher. The goal was to deny Bush and other lawmakers any applause for what the activists considered to be incremental improvements.

For example, in a May 2002 *New York Times* article that was otherwise congratulatory to members of Congress who had increased their attention to global AIDS, Dr. Paul Zeitz, executive director of the Global AIDS Alliance, wrote: "Three million Africans are going to die this year. I want $10 billion this year. I don't buy this incremental response. I think it's a hoax." When President Bush announced his 2002 Global Fund commitment of $200 million, OxFam America president Raymond C. Offenheiser told the *Washington Post,* "They left out a zero," and Health GAP

Coalition activists were quoted as saying the amount was "less than a drop in the bucket." More subtle media strategies included briefing editorial boards and supplying background information to reporters who attended global AIDS conferences and covered the visits to Africa by Colin Powell and other administration officials.

David Gartner of the Global AIDS Alliance cites all of these efforts in saying that O'Neill and others have underestimated the outside-the-White-House influence on PEPFAR. "You have to put the PEPFAR announcement in context," he says. "There was only one mention of Africa in the 2000 presidential debates, and the issue was not mentioned at all in that year's Republican Party platform. So it is not clear that Bush would have done anything at all but for the other people working on this—from Secretary-General Annan to Secretary Powell to activists, including evangelicals, along with members of Congress and the people doing pioneering AIDS treatment in the field."

But even Gartner says that this collective activist effort does not obscure the fact that it was the president who delivered that startlingly positive news from the podium on January 28, 2003. "To deny Bush credit for PEPFAR would be foolish," Gartner says. "He was not operating in a vacuum, but at the end of the day, he was the one who decided to take the bold step."

5

"WE ARE NOT A MORTUARY"

IN MID-2003, THE PEPFAR-INSPIRED hope in Washington had not yet reached the wards of Moi Teaching and Referral Hospital. There, a woman named Theresa huddled under a thin and tattered blanket in a bed she shared with another woman whose feet lay by Theresa's head. She looked up vacantly at the doctors and medical students surrounding her. Theresa was so thin—"wasted" was the term the Kenyan medical student used when reading aloud from his examination notes—that her eyes seemed to bulge out from above her sunken cheeks.

The medical student read on: Theresa had had a persistent cough for four years. Her breathing was rapid but shallow. Her mouth and throat were choked with a white fungus that made it seem as though Theresa had been chewing cotton. It was oral thrush, an indicator of AIDS. Theresa's breathing was so labored because she also had PCP—pneumocystis carinii pneumonia—one of the most common and serious infections for people with HIV.

The medical student closed by reciting the social history. Theresa was a twenty-eight-year-old widow with three children at home, the youngest just three years old. The student finished and looked up at Joe Mamlin, who was leading hospital rounds.

Mamlin shook his head and looked past the students toward a visitor from Indiana. "Unfortunately," he said, "that is your introduction to Kenya."

Mamlin then led the group on. Women lay two or even three to a bed, flies alighting on their heads. The physicians and students stepped around a woman curled up on the bare floor, clutching herself and moaning. They examined Elizabeth, who had arms the circumference of a broom handle. Janet was in a coma. Beatrice had skin lesions.

Alice hadn't been tested yet, but showed signs of late-stage HIV; she had lost her husband to the disease a few years before. One of the observers leaned over to read her hospital chart and was bumped in the hip by an attendant trying to maneuver a battered aluminum cart down the aisle. On the cart was a small body under a stained blanket. It was clear that, soon enough, all of these women would be on that cart.

But the next day, away from the grim Eldoret hospital wards, some signs of hope were beginning to emerge. At the Mosoriot Rural Health Center, twenty-five kilometers west of Eldoret, a young Kenyan woman walked into a closet-size room with concrete walls and pulled from a plastic bag three cardboard boxes, worn at the edges and dusted red by the region's clay soil. The woman handed the boxes to clinical officer Lillian Boit, who opened each box and counted the pills inside. The young woman was in perfect compliance with that month's triple therapy antiretroviral drug regimen. She had HIV, but she was healthy.

For five hours straight, Joe Mamlin sat next to Boit as patients came in one after another and Boit translated their Swahili or Nandi into English. Although told at first that their services were not needed in this community where no one said "HIV" aloud, the Indiana and Moi doctors had kept coming. For months, they treated other diseases and slowly built trust and relationships with the local residents. Now, twice a week, dozens of patients were openly acknowledging their HIV status by lining up to see Mamlin. Community groups were singing songs about HIV awareness, and a large sign advertising HIV testing was painted on the outside wall of the clinic.

The Mosoriot program was proving that rural Kenyans were quite able to comply with strict antiretroviral therapy, once widely thought to be unsuited to people living in the African countryside. Mamlin gestured to where Boit was explaining the requirements of the therapy to an HIV-positive pregnant woman whose husband had already agreed to get tested as well. "People say you can't do this in a village in Africa, but just look how intently they are paying attention to Lillian," he said. "This is life and death, and they know it. There is no doubt you can do this business out here."

Mosoriot's success as the first rural program for the Indiana–Moi team was due in no small part to the center's director, nurse Irene Kalamai. Kalamai's iron-fisted management of the center is matched by her personal compassion. She reveals her softer side often to clinic patients and on her own family farm, where she houses and feeds people whom she describes as "those whose heads are not very stable." Kalamai also supports various women in micro-enterprises selling herbal skin remedies, and she pays for some area orphans to attend secondary school in the city.

If rural Kenya is moving toward a more modern approach to gender roles, Irene Kalamai may represent the vanguard. Although her father had three wives (and thirty children), when Kalamai's husband brought another wife home, she walked out. "I said I could not stomach [it]," she says.

A member of the fiercely patriarchal Nandi ethnic group, Kalamai is equally ferocious in her determination to empower women medical professionals and the women who serve as traditional birth attendants throughout the countryside surrounding Mosoriot. Those women and Kalamai work in partnership with Indiana–Moi to provide education and treatment to pregnant women. "With the new drugs, we are not going to lose so many people," she says. "Widows now can be healthy and learn good farming so they do not always have to be dependent on aid. The men are now coming to be tested, which never used to happen. I tell them not to delay doing something until the person is so sick you have to carry them in. We are not a mortuary!"

By June 2003, AMPATH, now under the leadership of program manager Sylvester Kimaiyo, had reached its goal of treating 1,000 HIV patients. It was already Kenya's largest provider of HIV prevention and treatment services, and one of the most comprehensive HIV systems in the developing world. The Indiana and Moi physicians had jointly authored several research papers documenting their HIV control and treatment efforts, and those papers were starting to gain notice. "The IU–Moi model seeks to train Kenyan health care workers to be equipped to deal with the HIV/AIDS epidemic, which is critical if there is going to be any headway made," Dr. Marty Markowitz, clinical director of the New York–based Aaron Diamond AIDS Research Center, told an Indianapolis newspaper in 2003. "You cannot fight a war long-distance, you have to fight this war on the ground. And it can best be done by Kenyans, with the assistance of those more experienced."

Kimaiyo began being invited to conferences in Europe and Africa on HIV treatment, where he found himself inundated with questions about how Indiana–Moi had created and sustained its program. "One of the most remarkable things about the Indiana–Moi program is that they managed to get substantial numbers of patients on much-needed treatment well before factors like increased donor interest and reduced drug prices made decent treatment a reality in other settings in Kenya," Dr. Barbara Marston, of the Centers for Disease Control's Global AIDS Program, said in 2003. "As a result, they have capable care providers, well-established systems and the necessary buy-in from both the hospital administration and the community—and can therefore really ramp up in the face of these changes. Other programs are just now struggling to improve community awareness and provide the necessary training to health care personnel."

But, in 2003, a close look at even the successful outreach in Mosoriot showed the limits of the Indiana–Moi efforts. Dozens of women patients came to the clinic each week, all showing signs that their bodies were breaking down from the virus. PEPFAR funding had not hit the ground yet, and these women did not fit into any of the narrow categories—essentially pregnant women and their families—where Indiana–Moi had grant funding from the MTCT-Plus Initiative to provide antiretrovirals. For those who did not fit into this category, AMPATH could only prescribe antibiotics that helped temporarily fight off some of the secondary infections.

On that same day in 2003, just as Mamlin and Boit were finishing up their last patient at Mosoriot, a village man carried in his forty-two-year-old sister Evelyne, who was too weak to walk. Her heart rate was 161 sitting in a wheelchair, and she was fighting to get oxygen into her lungs. Evelyne was bundled up as if it were freezing outside, but her sleeves rode up to reveal painfully thin arms. Mamlin directed her brother to bring her to the Moi Teaching and Referral Hospital. After they left, Mamlin acknowledged that Evelyne had little chance of surviving the week. "For the 95 percent of patients we see who are not pregnant women, there is nothing for them here," he said. "Sometimes this is just hell."

❧

Even for the pregnant women Indiana–Moi was able to treat, difficult challenges remained. Without some sort of intervention, approximately one in every four HIV-positive mothers will transmit the virus to her child. In the initial years of AMPATH's efforts to prevent this transmission, the treatment protocol called for a single dose of the antiretroviral drug nevirapine provided at the outset of labor and a dose of nevirapine for the infant within forty-eight to seventy-two hours after delivery. For the many HIV-positive Kenyan mothers who chose to deliver at home or could not travel to a health clinic or hospital, AMPATH trained traditional birth attendants to provide the nevirapine.

But then researchers discovered that even the single dose of nevirapine provided to birthing mothers, while effective at preventing transmission of the virus to the baby, caused as many as two-thirds of the mothers to develop a resistance to the drug. This meant that nevirapine could not be used as a subsequent antiretroviral treatment for the mother. So AMPATH switched to the more complicated and expensive protocol of beginning full antiretroviral treatment for pregnant women in the twenty-eighth week of their pregnancy, and continuing on for two weeks after delivery.

An even thornier problem was presented after HIV-positive mothers gave birth. The medical consensus is that nutrition and antibodies in breast milk make it the best health option for infants, and breast-feeding is the cultural norm for Kenyan mothers. However, babies of HIV-positive mothers stand a substantial risk of contracting the virus from breast milk. For this reason, HIV-positive mothers in the U.S. and other developed nations are encouraged to forgo breast-feeding and feed their babies infant formula instead.

In Kenya and throughout the developing world, however, bacteria-laden water supplies can cause babies fed with formula mixed with water to contract deadly cases of diarrhea and respiratory infection. Formula-fed babies suffer from these illnesses at far higher rates than breast-fed babies who can avoid the dangerous water supply. A study of babies of HIV-positive mothers in Botswana, published in the *Journal of the American Medical Association* in 2006, found that breast-fed babies were more likely to contract HIV than formula-fed babies, but the formula-fed babies were more likely to die from other causes during their first year of life. However, an earlier study conducted in Nairobi, where HIV-positive mothers had access to a municipal water supply, found better outcomes for formula-fed babies.

Further complicating matters was the consensus that the most dangerous option for HIV-positive mothers is to combine breast-feeding and formula feeding. Formula feeding can irritate the lining of the baby's stomach and intestines, making it easier for HIV from the mother's milk to enter the bloodstream. Even when HIV-positive African mothers commit to exclusive formula feeding, cultural stigma or unreliable supplies of formula can pressure them to mix in breast-feeding.

After weighing all the imperfect options, AMPATH settled on a strategy of having frank discussions with HIV-positive mothers about their ability to commit themselves to feeding their baby solely with formula, and to provide both formula and water purification systems to mothers who could make the commitment. But problems with maintaining clean water and an uninterrupted formula supply, and with ensuring that mothers were thoroughly cleaning bottles, led AMPATH to alter its recommended procedures in 2007. The new preferred protocol called for giving pregnant mothers an option of formula feeding or taking anti-retroviral drugs before delivery and until the baby was weaned, in the not completely confirmed hope that the medicine would lower the risk of transmission without harming the baby.

To Bob Einterz, the difficulty of finding the appropriate pro-cedure for feeding babies born to HIV-positive mothers in Kenya illustrates the challenge of practicing medicine, especially in Af-rica. "Medicine is science-based," he says, "but at the end of the day, the practice of medicine is an art. People in the U.S. expect so much certainty in medicine, and expect their doctors to do just the right thing. But all you have is the evidence at hand. And that evidence will be augmented next week and the next month and the next year. In Africa in particular, and with a sensitive issue like breast-feeding in particular, it shows that health is not just science or medicine, it is as much a question of politics and economics and culture."

Before and after the PEPFAR announcement, the focus in both Washington and Africa was firmly on delivering lifesaving treat-ment to the HIV-infected population. But Mamlin and Kimaiyo were discovering that, even for the lucky few they could provide with antiretrovirals, the medicine was sometimes not enough. In April 2002, thirty-four-year-old Salina Rotich was carried into the Mosoriot clinic, weighing only seventy-three pounds and suffering from tuberculosis and PCP as a result of AIDS. Mamlin treated her pneumonia and TB and put her on antiretrovirals, looking forward to seeing Rotich at follow-up visits enjoying the legendary "Lazarus effect" of the medicine.

But when she came back in to the clinic two weeks later, Rotich was still very sick and wasted, and seemed even closer to death. A startled Mamlin began asking her questions about her home situation, and discovered that she was eating virtu-ally nothing. Like many of AMPATH's women patients, Salina Rotich had already lost her husband to AIDS before she sought treatment, and now she herself was too weak with illness to tend her small farm or seek other work. Mamlin began giving Rotich a few Kenyan shillings to buy cornmeal, milk, and eggs. Immediately, her health began to improve. Within six months, Rotich had doubled her body weight and had returned to caring for her five children and tending two acres of maize.

It turned out that Salina Rotich's hunger was not uncommon. As he and Kimaiyo saw more and more HIV-positive patients, Mamlin discovered that as many as one in five of them did not have enough food. Malnutrition was blunting the effect of the antiretrovirals, and the side effects of taking the medicine on empty stomachs were interfering with patient compliance with the drug regimen. "Around this time, I visited the UN World Food Program's operation in Busia near here, and I saw they were feeding thirty-six thousand people," Mamlin says. "But after some short-term health gains from being fed, HIV-infected people were getting weaker again because no one was treating their disease. Here, we were doing the opposite: giving the drugs but no food. And I saw the mirror image of WFP's problem with our patients: the drugs were not enough because they were hungry.

"When it comes down to it, HIV is poverty. We simply had to get in the business of reconstituting not just immune systems, but the patients' entire lives."

So Mamlin persuaded the Mosoriot high school to donate an unused ten-acre parcel of land. He then hired Steve Lewis, a Welsh farmer who was already helping develop community farms in the area, to launch AMPATH into the farming business. Soon, AMPATH patients who needed nutrition support were given "prescriptions" for food, which were filled with vegetables, milk, and eggs raised at AMPATH farms, along with maize, beans, and cooking oil from the World Food Program. Like Salina Rotich, most patients were supporting other family members, so they were given enough food for their dependents as well. Six months on this food regimen turned out to be enough for most patients to benefit from the reconstitution of their immune system and, hopefully, return to self-sufficiency. By the end of 2007, AMPATH was feeding thirty thousand people each week.

But for some patients, like Evelyne Njoki, poverty and HIV stigma still blocked the road to self-sufficiency. Njoki grew up as one of six children who lived with their parents in a two-room house in a slum in the town of Nanyuki, just a few kilometers from the equator. Her family could not afford school fees, so she left school at age sixteen. In 2002, Njoki was pregnant and had just moved to Eldoret with the father of the child, a man also from Nanyuki, when a prenatal exam revealed that she was HIV-positive. She urged the father to get tested as well. Instead, he left Njoki and returned to Nanyuki, leaving her pregnant and with no source of support.

With the help of AMPATH treatment, Njoki delivered a healthy HIV-negative baby, a girl named Wanjiru. But she and the baby struggled to find food and a place to live. "I could not go back home to my family because of my status," she said, referring to the stigma of being HIV-positive. She received some food support from the local Catholic archdiocese, but she was being threatened with eviction from her rented room, had no land to farm, and no prospects for a job.

Njoki did have a knack for handcrafts, though, and began to go room to room at Moi Teaching and Referral Hospital selling beads and ribbons she had made. Her entrepreneurial efforts attracted the attention of Benjamin Andama and Peter Park, co-directors of a new AMPATH program called Family Preservation Initiative, designed to help patients support themselves. (AMPATH's management structure copied the U.S. Peace Corps model of counterpart relationships. Just as Kimaiyo and Mamlin jointly led AMPATH overall, the Kenyan Andama and the American Park were installed as co-directors of the effort to promote income self-sufficiency.)

Njoki persuaded Andama and Park to loan her 9,000 Kenyan shillings (about $150 U.S.) to buy wholesale beads from Nairobi. She began making necklaces from the beads at night and taking baby Wanjiru with her to sell them during the day. Njoki repaid the loan, and soon was making a good living selling her personally crafted jewelry. Eventually, she agreed to Andama and Park's request that she leave her business behind to begin training other AMPATH patients in bead making. Within a few months, Njoki was helping direct the new Imani Workshop ("imani" means faith in Kiswahili), where AMPATH patients made jewelry and sewed handbags and clothing. First a handful, then a few hundred, and ultimately thousands of AMPATH patients came to Imani to follow Njoki's lead in learning to support themselves and their families. "I'm able to pay my house rent, I'm able to get my daily bread," Njoki says now. "At first, I was feeling so hopeless but for now, life has changed. I'm stable, and at first I was seeing as if I'm dying, but now I'm hoping to live."

6

CAN FOREIGN
AID WORK?

IN HIS POWERPOINT PRESENTATIONS to U.S. groups, Bob Einterz likes
to show a photo of a truck labeled "Kenya AIDS Control Pro-
gramme"—crushed from the top down and abandoned in the
weeds. It seemed a perfect metaphor for the recent decades' efforts
to control disease and poverty in Africa. Haroun arap Mengech
had seen ambitious foreign-funded health programs founder in
Kenya, partly because aid money was misdirected once it landed
within the country. As AMPATH began to expand, both in its
number of HIV-positive patients treated and in the scope of services provided, its leaders were well aware they were operating
in a venue filled with failed aid efforts.

Despite the accolades greeting President Bush's 2003 PEPFAR
announcement, foreign aid in Africa and the developing world
had a checkered reputation, with some reason. William Easterly,
a former World Bank economist who moved on to become a professor at New York University, points out that a whopping $568
billion in 2007 dollars had been delivered as aid to Africa since
1965, yet the per capita economic growth of those recipient African nations has been close to zero. Even after all those billions,

the continent overall was just as poor as it had been when the influx of aid began.

In multiple articles and speeches and in his 2006 book, *The White Man's Burden: How the West's Efforts to Aid the Rest Have Done So Much Ill and So Little Good,* Easterly cites economic studies showing that foreign aid does not help a struggling nation. In fact, Easterly argues, aid actually reduces the prospects for democracy and rule of law and increases the likelihood of corruption. "Large aid flows can result in a reduction in government accountability because governing elites no longer need to ensure the support of their publics and assent of their legislatures when they do not need revenues from the local economy," he wrote in a 2007 article. Easterly also ridicules the bureaucracy of foreign aid, pointing out that his former employer the World Bank has ten thousand employees and that a struggling country like Tanzania has to issue 2,400 different reports each year to satisfy aid donors. Among the commentators who agree with Easterly is Nicolas van de Walle, a Michigan State University professor. In his 2001 book, *African Economies and the Politics of Permanent Crisis,* van de Walle argued that by sustaining ineffective policies that otherwise would have been corrected by market forces, aid has blocked the chances for needed changes in dysfunctional African countries.

Easterly, van de Walle, and other aid critics focus on this market-distorting effect of foreign development assistance, which they say stifles homegrown political and economic reforms. (Only partly tongue-in-cheek, Easterly claims that Lenin was the twentieth century's first development economist.) Easterly argues that recent economic development success stories like China, India, and Chile have occurred only after donors and experts got out of the way of indigenous leadership. "The only 'answer' to poverty reduction is freedom from being told the answer," Easterly wrote in "Freeing the Poor," an article published in the periodical *Foreign Policy* in 2007. "Free societies and individuals are not guaranteed to be saved. They will make bad choices. But at least they will bear the cost of those mistakes, and learn from them."

Paul Collier, an Oxford professor and like Easterly a former World Bank official, is not as strenuous a critic of foreign aid, but he is convinced that aid is not adequate to the task of lifting the world's poorest people out of poverty. Aid must be supplemented by action, including military interventions and targeted trade policies, Collier says in his 2007 book, *The Bottom Billion: Why the Poorest Countries Are Failing and What Can Be Done about It*. "With some important exceptions, aid does not work so well in these environments, at least as it has been provided in the past," Collier writes. "Change in these societies at the very bottom must come predominately from within; we cannot impose it on them."

HIV/AIDS assistance is singled out for specific criticism by Helen Epstein, a microbiologist and AIDS activist, in her 2007 book, *The Invisible Cure: Africa, the West, and the Fight against AIDS*. Epstein criticizes donor countries pushing abstinence and condoms on Africans, and notes that even ambitious treatment efforts like PEPFAR and the Global Fund to Fight HIV/AIDS, Tuberculosis, and Malaria are only treating a fraction of the continent's HIV-infected population. Like others who have studied HIV in sub-Saharan Africa, Epstein concludes that the common African practice of having concurrent long-term sexual partners is the key to explaining the wildfire spread of the disease. Curbing that concurrent partner habit, Epstein argues, is the "invisible cure" for the pandemic and was the key factor in Uganda's dramatic drop in HIV prevalence from 30 percent of adults in 1992 to less than 10 percent in 2003. (It should be noted that there are a host of competing explanations for Uganda's unparalleled statistical success, including a possible original overcount of HIV prevalence, the intervening death of so many infected Ugandans, and the impact of an aggressive condom and safe-sex marketing campaign.)

Echoing Easterly's premise that local initiative is the only solution to African crises, Epstein says this invisible cure was accomplished more by local efforts than by any foreign help. "[Ugandan president] Yoweri Museveni's government developed its own vigorous prevention campaigns and the World Health Organization provided funding, but much also came from the poor themselves," Epstein writes. "Their compassion and hard work brought the disease into the open, got people talking about the epidemic, reduced AIDS-related stigma and denial, and led to a shift in sexual norms."

Epstein concludes that western involvement with the AIDS fight in Africa is often so misdirected and self-serving that it diverts valuable resources from local programs that hold more promise for curbing the disease. Like Easterly, Epstein says that large aid organizations receiving support from PEPFAR, the Bill and Melinda Gates Foundation, or the Global Fund are often too focused on generating reports that will impress the bureaucracies that control their funding. This obsession with reporting the numbers of people served can lead to situations like the one described in the chilling indictment from the founder of a South African AIDS orphan program, who told Epstein, "When the Americans come, we sing, we dance, they take our picture, and they go back and show everyone how they are helping the poor black people. But then all they do is hijack our projects and count our children."

Epstein notes that as foreign AIDS spending rose sharply in Uganda after 2000, bringing with it hundreds of representatives of aid agencies, the HIV rate stopped its decline. "It is possible that as the response to AIDS became bureaucratized by foreign aid, and as informal efforts morphed into 'strategic frameworks,' 'operational plans,' 'workplace issues,' and 'focal points'—all with vast budgets—the critical human element, without which no development program in Africa can possibly succeed, was lost," she writes.

Even if the historically high amount of foreign aid focused on the HIV/AIDS pandemic is more successful in fighting the disease than Epstein believes it will be, it still may not be enough. Others say that PEPFAR and the Global Fund, not to mention the work of the Gates Foundation and high-profile celebrity activists like Bono, are too focused on a few diseases like HIV, tuberculosis, and malaria. By obscuring the broader health challenges of the developing world, these well-meaning actors could actually worsen global poverty, says Laurie Garrett, a noted international health journalist and author of *Betrayal of Trust: The Collapse of Global Health*. In an early 2007 issue of the influential periodical *Foreign Affairs*, Garrett wrote that contributions by PEPFAR, the Global Fund, and the Gates Foundation to eradicating disease are "mind-boggling," but also largely misguided.

"One would think that with all this money on the table, the solutions to many global health problems would at least now be in sight," Garrett wrote. "But one would be wrong." According to Garrett, the effectiveness of these well-funded antidisease efforts is hampered by a decentralized and uncoordinated approach to care. She estimates there are over sixty thousand AIDS-related non-governmental organizations (NGOs) alone, with even more devoted to general global health. In addition, corruption and bureaucracy siphon off huge chunks of aid money before it ever reaches the patients. A 2006 World Bank report reached the disturbing conclusion that nearly half of all donated funds for sub-Saharan African health efforts never reached the care providers in clinics and hospitals. Worse than mere inefficiency, Garrett argues that disease-specific programs with bulging budgets can seduce scarce professional medical talent away from developing countries' broader health systems. Those systems already suffer from a profound "brain drain" when health professionals leave their home countries for better-paying work in North America and western Europe.

Garrett says the new global health programs funded by PEP-FAR and the Gates Foundation don't build the developing countries' capacity to eventually lead and sustain their own health-care efforts. "Nearly all [programs] have been designed, managed and executed by residents of the wealthy world," she writes. "Virtually no provisions exist to allow the world's poor to say what they want, decide which projects serve their needs, or adopt local innovations."

Garrett's prescription for change is to switch the global health focus away from HIV/AIDS and other disease-specific programming to broader health-care system improvement. Of course, the push toward disease-specific programs came about in part because more broadly focused forms of aid had proven hard to monitor and were often subject to waste and misuse. But Garrett insists that improvement in broader health systems can be precisely measured by increased maternal survival rate and increased life expectancy. Those indicators, she says, reflect both a well-funded health-care delivery system and successful public health programs that ensure safe water, immunizations, and adequate food supply. To Garrett, those general improvements through local initiatives are the only sustainable form of success. "For the day will come," she writes, "when the charity eases off and programs collapse, and unless workable local institutions have already been established, little will remain to show for all of the current frenzied activity."

❊

The existing efforts to combat HIV/AIDS, malaria, and tuberculosis, along with other, wider aid-focused development efforts, have their own champions, of course. With the possible exception of the high-wattage Bono, Jeffrey Sachs, Columbia University economics professor and UN special adviser, is the most ubiquitous proponent of aggressive aid programs. In his 2005 book, ambitiously titled *The End of Poverty,* Sachs outlined confident assertions that the UN Millennium Development Goals—universal primary education, improved maternal health, and reductions in child poverty, HIV/AIDS, and other diseases—are readily achievable. But it will take continued and increased aid to get there, Sachs writes. "Until Africa's economies pull Africa out of extreme poverty—something that will be powerfully assisted by disease control—foreign aid is not a whim, a matter of dole, or a matter of avoidable dependency. It is a matter of life and death. We have just started on the road to doing this, after decades of shocking neglect."

Sachs acknowledges "the widespread belief that aid is simply wasted money down the rat hole" and concedes that there are many examples of failed aid programs, which are often tainted by the donor countries' political motivations. "But these notorious cases obscure the critical fact that development assistance based on proven technologies and directed at measurable and practical needs—increased food production, disease control, safe water and sanitation, schoolrooms and clinics, Internet connectivity and the like—has a distinguished record of success." As part of his proof, Sachs points to steady and significant increases in life expectancy in poorer countries, especially before the AIDS pandemic began to undo that progress.

Sachs is known for chiding the United States and other western democracies for foreign aid commitments that appear minuscule next to other government expenditures. Most pointedly, he notes that a full year's worth of current U.S. aid to Africa is equal to less than three days' worth of U.S. military spending. Sachs predicts that the agricultural "Green Revolution" that helped raise India out of famine to relative prosperity can be replicated in Africa, but says that targeted disease-control programs, along with fertilizer and high-yield seed support for farmers, will be necessary to allow Africans to be healthy and prepared to pull themselves out of poverty. "We need more aid, not aid bashing," Sachs writes.

By most accounts, the early results of PEPFAR have provided support for the argument that well-planned foreign aid can make a large and positive impact on the lives of Africa's poor. In December 2008, the U.S. Office of the Global AIDS Coordinator announced that PEPFAR had now placed more than two million HIV-positive patients on antiretroviral treatment in the program's fifteen focus countries, and provided services to more than six million pregnant women to prevent mother-to-child transmission of HIV. In more than a half million of those cases, the women were found to be HIV-positive and received antiretroviral drugs to prevent infant infections. PEPFAR had supported care for nearly four million children left orphaned or vulnerable by AIDS, and paid for 57 million HIV counseling and testing sessions for men, women, and children.

The Institute of Medicine, the branch of the National Academies that had been directed by Congress to deliver an independent three-year report card on PEPFAR, issued positive findings in March 2007. "The Committee concludes that PEPFAR has made a good start toward meeting [its] targets and establishing the program to make further progress . . . The first three years of PEPFAR have been characterized by a sense of urgency and by rapid implementation of programs."

Activists often criticize PEPFAR's mandate that abstinence-until-marriage programs account for one-third of the program's prevention spending, and they oppose PEPFAR's preference for purchasing brand-name drugs over cheaper generic products.

But every major global health advocacy group supported President Bush's 2007 proposal to reauthorize PEPFAR for five more years and double the U.S. investment to $30 billion during that period. In fact, as of this writing in early 2008, many members of Congress are supporting a significantly larger increase in funding—to $50 billion. When Republican senator Richard Lugar of Indiana introduced the Senate legislation to renew PEPFAR, he said, "Five years ago, HIV was a death sentence for most individuals in the developing world who contracted the disease. Now there is hope. We should never forget that behind each number is a person—a life the United States can touch or even save." It was a sentiment echoed on both sides of the political aisle.

Warren "Buck" Buckingham, the veteran U.S. HIV/AIDS activist who is now the Kenya country coordinator for PEPFAR, says he and other program leaders have learned that there are significant challenges to providing services in sub-Saharan Africa, including the need for infrastructure, safe water, and security for drug inventory. "But the triumph is that we learned that all it takes is money to fix these things," he says. "The human will can be mobilized to accomplish great things. In Kenya, we went from three very small pilot programs in 2002, where we were treating only 342 people in all, to where we are now in mid-2007, putting 340-plus more people on antiretrovirals every day."

Buckingham says that over a hundred thousand Kenyans are now receiving antiretroviral medicine at 280 sites supported by PEPFAR. "This should put to an end to any argument about 'absorptive capacity,' the idea that if you put massive amounts of resources into a developing country's health crisis, you just create massive opportunities for corruption and graft. PEPFAR has demonstrated that, with rigorous monitoring and oversight, you actually get what you are paying for."

Nana Poku, director of research for the Commission on HIV/AIDS and Governance in Africa, a UN initiative, echoed Buckingham's assessment in his 2005 book *AIDS in Africa: How the Poor Are Dying*. Poku reviewed the record of an aggressive antiretroviral therapy program operated by Médecins Sans Frontières (Doctors Without Borders) in Khayelitsha township in Cape Town, South Africa. "[The Khayelitsha program] suggests strongly that scaling up treatment is feasible and that this can be accomplished through a focus on expanding access to antiretroviral therapy and related services to the primary care level," Poku concluded. "It is possible to achieve very favourable outcomes in terms of reduced morbidity and mortality, so that individuals, families and communities can manage the personal and social impact of HIV/AIDS."

The Center for Global Development, based in Washington, D.C., responded to the debate about the effectiveness of foreign aid by convening a "What Works Working Group" of experts in global health, economics, and public policy. Led by Ruth Levine, senior fellow at the center and its vice president for programs and operations, the group reviewed large-scale efforts to improve health in developing countries and published its findings in the book *Millions Saved: Proven Success in Global Health.* The report outlines twenty cases, including the vaccination campaigns that led to the nearly total elimination of measles as a cause of childhood death in southern Africa, the condom program that led to an 80 percent reduction in HIV cases among high-risk populations in Thailand, and safe-motherhood services in Sri Lanka that sharply reduced maternal mortality. "This work provides clear evidence that large-scale success in health is possible—countering a common view that the health problems of the developing world are intractable, and that development assistance to health yields few benefits," the working group concluded.

In fact, a closer review of the positions staked out by foreign aid critics like William Easterly (who is a nonresident fellow at the Center for Global Development, which sponsors the What Works Working Group) shows grudging support for aid directed to programs that focus on public health and basic services. In *White Man's Burden,* Easterly acknowledges foreign aid's role in spurring dramatic improvements in health and education in poor countries. He delivers explicit approval for continuing the kind of aid that forms the core of the Millennium Development Goals he routinely criticizes. "[We should] get the poorest people in the world such obvious goods as the vaccines, the antibiotics, the roads, the boreholes, the water pipes, the textbooks, the nurses. This is not making the poor dependent on handouts; it is giving the poorest people the health, nutrition, education and other inputs that raise the payoff to their own efforts to better their lives." Van de Walle and other foreign aid critics make similar concessions to the fact that emergency health aid has undeniably eased suffering throughout Africa.

Given this extensive laundry list of "acceptable" foreign aid provided by aid's most vocal opponents, and the fact that aid advocates like Sachs admit that donations have often been dismally managed, it appears there may not be as much controversy over foreign aid as is implied by harsh op-ed rhetoric and provocative book titles. Indeed, Helen Epstein and Laurie Garrett have responded to their critics by stating that it is not foreign aid itself that they oppose, just the habitually unwise method in which it is provided.

Ultimately, few experts truly disagree with the concept that western governments should directly help the poor and sick people of Africa. But their support for aid is contingent on programs avoiding the common pitfalls of bureaucracy and corruption, while at the same time empowering local leadership and building capacity for long-term indigenous success. Achieving that balance is far easier said than done, but as PEPFAR began to roll out in 2004 and 2005, AMPATH was earning a reputation as a program that was pulling off this difficult feat in western Kenya.

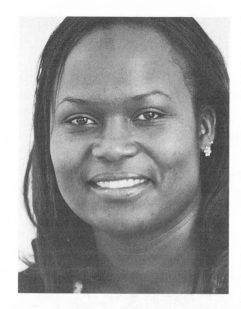

Figure 18. (left) In the midst of a violent conflict in early 2007, Dr. Caroline Kosgei defied police evacuation orders to stay in the besieged AMPATH Mt. Elgon clinic and treat her patients. PHOTO BY FRAN QUIGLEY.

Figure 19. (below) John Nandi of Bindura, Kenya, is the grandfather of these children and has been their sole caretaker since their parents died of HIV/AIDS. AMPATH helped provide school uniforms for the children and fertilizer and seeds for planting the small farm of this family, which is one of thousands assisted by AMPATH's program for orphans and vulnerable children. PHOTO BY TOMEKA PETERSEN.

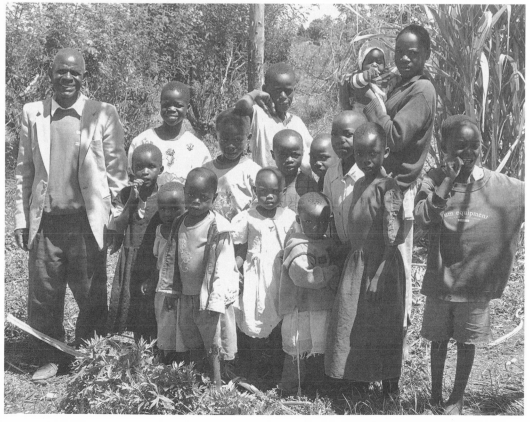

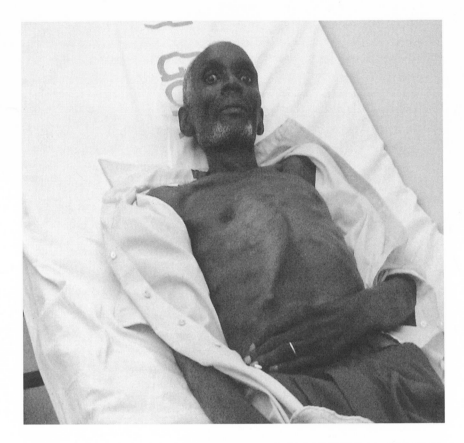

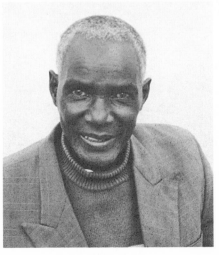

Figures 20 and 21. Musa Masudi Andinga came into the AMPATH clinic severely wasted, but therapeutic feeding and antiretroviral treatment returned him to robust health.

Photos by Joe Mamlin.

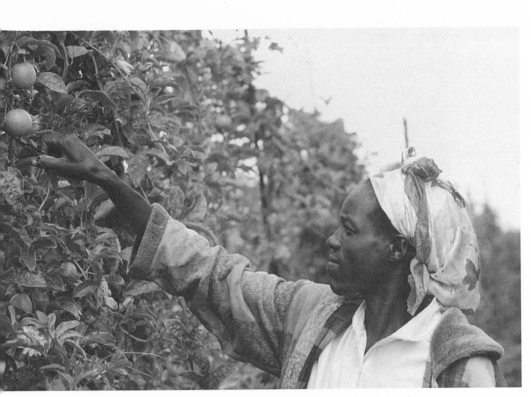

Figure 22. Irene Cheboi is one of many AMPATH patients now supporting their families by raising passion fruit on their small farms in the western Kenya highlands. Cheboi received seedlings and expert support through the AMPATH farming cooperative called Amkatwende, which is Kiswahili for "rise up, we go."

PHOTO BY FRAN QUIGLEY.

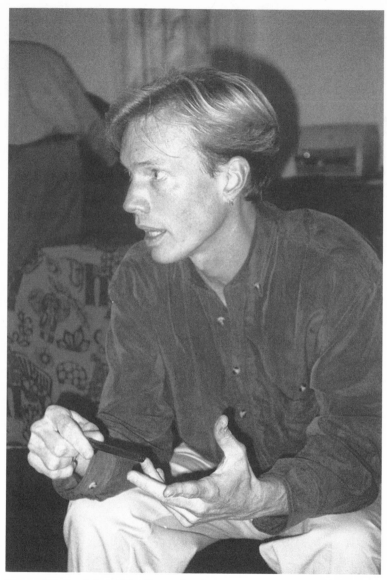

Figure 23. Dr. John Sidle directed Indiana University's program in Kenya during the most desperate of times for HIV patients, then returned to provide antiretroviral care and create a substance abuse counseling program for patients.
PHOTO BY FRAN QUIGLEY.

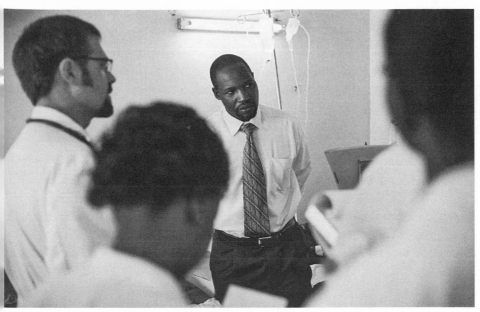

Figure 24. Moi University professor Dr. A. M Siika leads hospital rounds with Kenyan and U.S. medical students.
PHOTO BY TYAGAN MILLER.

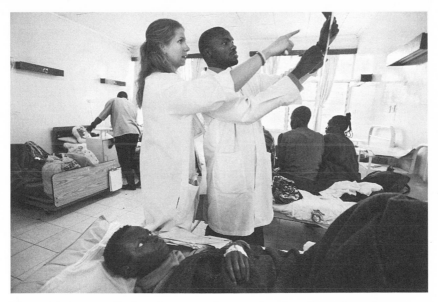

Figure 25. Two medical students, one from Moi University and one from Indiana University, examine a patient's x-rays at Moi Teaching and Referral Hospital.
PHOTO BY TYAGAN MILLER.

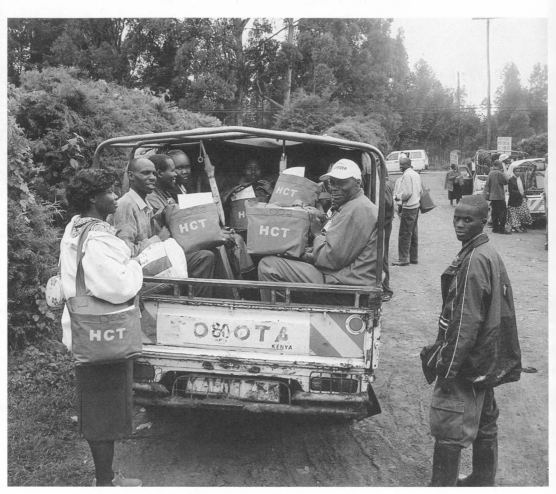

Figure 26. Home-based counseling and testing (HCT) moves AMPATH's response to the HIV/AIDS pandemic "upstream" to reach the Kenyan people before the virus has spread widely.

Photo by Tyagan Miller.

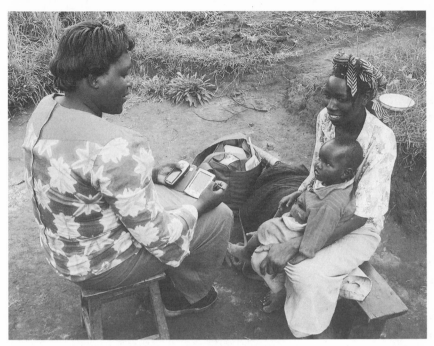

Figure 27. The HCT program uses advanced technology, including personal data assistants (PDAs) and global positioning system (GPS) receivers, to accurately track patients' history and the prevalence of HIV in rural Kenyan communities.

Photo by Tyagan Miller.

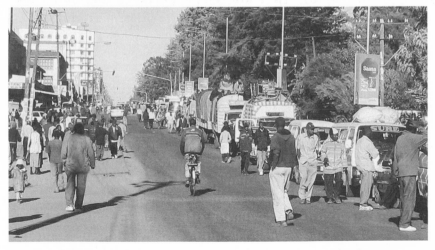

Figure 28. Postelection violence in early 2008 forced thousands of Kenyans from the Kikuyu ethnic group to leave western Kenya.

Photo by Joe Mamlin.

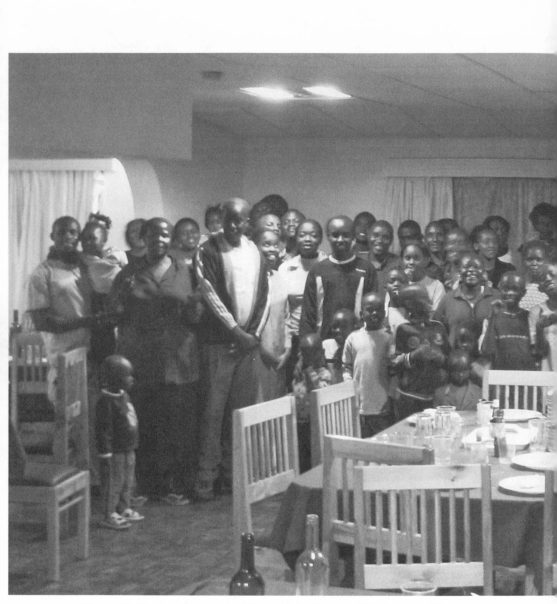

Figure 29. During the worst of the postelection conflict, dozens of Kenyans found sanctuary in the Indiana University compound in Eldoret.
PHOTO BY JOE MAMLIN.

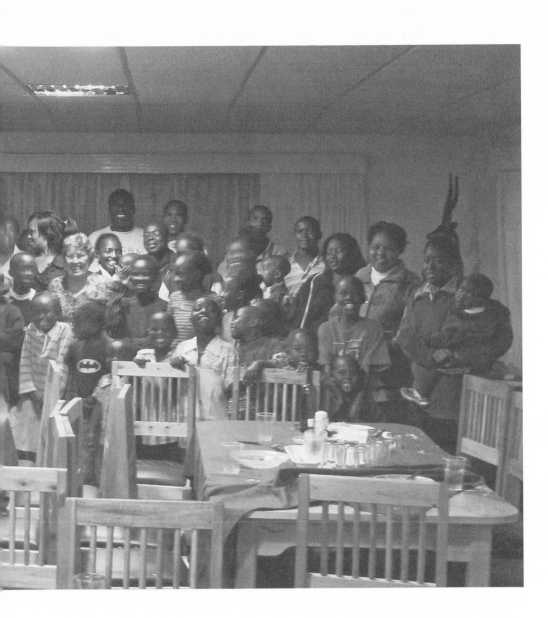

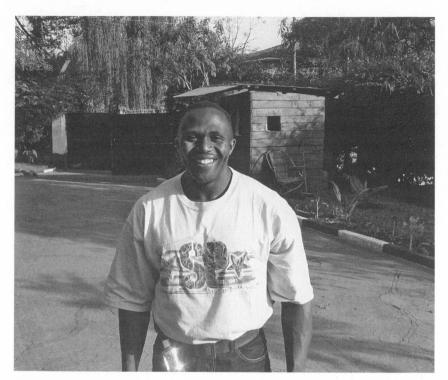

Figure 30. AMPATH staffer Javan Odinga risked his own life to deliver students from a different ethnic group to safety. During the postelection conflict in early 2008, Odinga was one of many AMPATH staffers who ignored both personal risk and ethnic differences to help fellow Kenyans. Photo by Joe Mamlin.

7

THE POWER OF THE ACADEMIC HEALTH CENTER

EVEN FOREIGN AID CRITICS CONCEDE that health initiatives in developing countries are worthy efforts, and aid supporters admit that far too many well-intentioned programs have failed miserably. The next question is what type of global health program can succeed. The "What Works" group of the Center for Global Development identified elements shared by successful large-scale global health programs; these included predictable and adequate funding, good management, and effective partnerships.

PEPFAR's Buck Buckingham says that Indiana–Moi had strong management and partnership in place by 2004, allowing AMPATH to seize on the suddenly plentiful PEPFAR funding. "There are two approaches to take when dealing with a global health crisis like AIDS," Buckingham says. "Too often, organizations will take the first approach, which is to set up an absolutely perfect teeny tiny timid project. What sets AMPATH apart is that it immediately took the second approach, which is to recognize that people are dying, and we got to get the treatment to them ASAP. That kind of 'just do it' attitude takes dynamic leadership, which AMPATH clearly has with Joe Mamlin.

"What also makes AMPATH unique is that it is a true partnership. It avoids the donor-recipient dynamic, because each partner has real value to contribute to the work being done. I've seen other university partnerships struggle to get beyond research, and too often the American partner to an African institution wants everything to happen in a twenty-four- to thirty-six-month grant timeline. Things just don't happen that way, especially in the developing world. So part of the challenge is to encourage long-term thinking."

Dr. Jean Lebel of the Ontario-based International Development Research Centre, an expert on health and research partnerships between the global north and the global south, agrees that the challenge of relationships like Indiana and Moi's lies in adapting expectations about what health programs can achieve. "We northerners tend to go to the south and try to simply replicate what we have done in our home settings," Lebel says. "But the infrastructure may be limited in the global south, and the programs that match what we are doing in the north may not exist at all.

"The secret to success lies in the ability of the two partners to learn from each other, and maintain an equilibrium so that one partner is not dominating the scheme, which has a lot to do with respect and trust. If that can be achieved, both partners have the ability to go beyond their usual boundaries."

Sylvester Kimaiyo acknowledges that it has not always been easy for Indiana and Moi to maintain a balance in their relationship. "There are clearly cultural differences," Kimaiyo says. "The people from IU [Indiana University] are a little faster and more aggressive in things like publishing papers, which can lead to them overrunning our Kenyan colleagues. So we responded by requiring that Americans publishing papers out of AMPATH try to include Kenyan counterparts in all of their work. Also, in the AMPATH management structure, from the very top to areas like community mobilization or economic self-sufficiency, we have set it up so that every leadership role is filled with a Kenyan and U.S. counterpart."

With personnel and expertise flowing into Kenya from Indiana University, the Kenyan medical community is the most obvious beneficiary of the partnership. But program participants from both countries are quick to point out that Indiana enjoys significant benefits as well. Hundreds of Indiana medical students and doctors in the Indiana University–Wishard Memorial Hospital network have spent time in Kenya, and they often return from the experience with valuable exposure to the treatment of infectious diseases and more sensitive to the impact of lifestyle and poverty on the health of their patients.

Dr. Ben Wince, an Indiana University School of Medicine graduate, says his Kenya experience made him a better doctor. "Dr. Einterz swears that Kenya is the best place to learn medicine, and I know what he means now," Wince says. "I had a college background in biomedical engineering, and I used to think technology was everything. But the experience in Kenya, where literally all you have is patient history and an examination, forced me to learn that you need to treat the whole person, not just the disease. What I know now is that sometimes technology can interfere with the doctor-patient relationship." Wince and other students and faculty also express admiration for Moi University's models of problem-based medical education and the Kenyan school's emphasis on learning through community-based research and practice in underserved rural areas.

To the leaders of AMPATH, the secret of the program's success in confronting the HIV/AIDS pandemic lies in the fact that the two institutions in partnership are academic health centers. The term "academic health center"—or the previously more common term "academic medical center"—is applied to a variety of different organizations. As the CEO of one such center told the Brookings Institution for a 2000 study, "If you've seen one academic medical center, you've seen one academic medical center." But all academic health centers do share a three-part mission: (1) training physicians and possibly other health-care providers in classroom and clinical care settings; (2) conducting research activities in laboratory and/or clinical settings; and (3) providing care in hospital and/or outpatient settings.

Academia enjoys immense power and prestige in both the developed and the developing world. But there are often questions about whether the academic community is able to or interested in effectively mobilizing its assets to tackle social problems. The twentieth-century philosopher Isaiah Berlin once said that the trouble with academics is that they are more concerned about whether ideas are interesting than whether they are true. Even if that is true of academics in general, it does not apply well to the clinical education model of academic medicine. Since U.S. medical students begin clinical rotations after just two years of classroom instruction, and professors engage in active medical practices of their own, any affection for interesting but false theories can be fatal to their patients.

Similarly, there is no other academic model parallel to academic medicine's widespread commitment to providing direct services for the poor and underserved. A study published in a 1996 issue of the journal *Academic Medicine* showed that low-income persons and/or those belonging to ethnic minorities constituted the majority of patients cared for in U.S. urban academic health centers. The same study showed that the academic health centers were taking on a disproportionate share of patients in their region who were completely unable to pay for care.

AMPATH's leadership says that academic health centers' combination of institutional resources and commitment to training, research, and care puts them in the ideal position to tackle the health-care crises of the developing world. While trying to bolster the shaky Nangrahar University medical school in Jalalabad back in 1967, Joe Mamlin repeatedly wrote to his Indiana University colleagues urging a more formal relationship with the Afghan institution. "I grew up professionally understanding there is power in the academic health center," Mamlin says now. "I watched it do its magic in Indianapolis [where Wishard Memorial Hospital and Indiana University created a system of neighborhood-based primary health care centers] and I saw it start to do important things in Afghanistan. Even though we weren't able to sustain the affiliation there, Afghanistan helped me discover the power of an academic health center to help those who are left out. There is a goodness in the academic medical center, so you want to move it to the depths of its creativity."

African academic health centers like Moi University School of Medicine and Moi Teaching and Referral Hospital are nowhere near as well funded and technologically advanced as U.S. academic health centers. But Sylvester Kimaiyo and Haroun arap Mengech say they have similar potential. "I've been in both the position of the dean of the medical school and director of the teaching hospital," Mengech says. "And from those vantage points, I can see quite clearly the value of the research, the training, and the care. Each one enriches the other." In a 2007 issue of the journal *Academic Medicine*, Einterz, Mengech, Kimaiyo, and Mamlin co-authored an article, "Responding to the HIV Pandemic: The Power of an Academic Medical Partnership," in which they insisted that academic health centers were in fact "the only resource in the U.S. and Africa capable of simultaneously providing service, mobilizing manpower, teaching and conducting research."

"The challenge of the HIV/AIDS pandemic and the other health crises in Africa fits perfectly into the tripartite care, training, and research mission of academic health centers," Einterz says. "First and foremost, the task is to understand what the problem is, which academic health centers can do because they confront it every day in delivering services. Then it is necessary to study the problem with research, followed by teaching the solutions to the providers. Then the loop is again closed by implementing the solutions through care. There is no other entity besides academic health centers that can do all that."

But even if all of the African, North American, and European academic health centers agreed tomorrow to band together to respond to the HIV/AIDS pandemic, Einterz and his AMPATH colleagues agree that a shift would first be necessary in the typical pecking order for the three goals of research, training, and care. "The tradition of academic health centers often emphasizes research and training," Einterz says. "Research, especially, is what is funded, and faculty promotions are judged on research publications. That is the bottom line."

AMPATH's leaders and other global health advocates say that elevating research to a position of primacy can limit the potential of a North–South academic health center partnership. In the 1990s, a major U.S. university came to Eldoret with funding to do research on sexually transmitted diseases, an important issue then and now. "But their focus, as best as I could tell, was only on doing research," Einterz says. "So they moved in with a lot of money to do the research and we saw faculty members from Moi University School of Medicine, which was already struggling because it had so few faculty, fleeing from clinics and the classrooms into the research project and research meetings, because that was where the dollars were.

"If this U.S university had worked to put their research project in context of the overall care and training missions of the school, they could have leveraged their research to the betterment of the health system as a whole. I'm not suggesting that research itself is not of value—this research on STDs was certainly of value. But they ended up focusing on research to the detriment of the health-care and training system as a whole. And we see this over and over and over again. It is commonly referred to as 'internal brain drain,' where the best and brightest medical minds get sucked off into the high-paying jobs of NGOs [non-governmental organizations]."

So Mamlin, Kimaiyo, Mengech, and Einterz adopted the philosophy that the Indiana–Moi partnership would honor the academic health centers' tripartite mission, but would lead with care. "We always hold high the banner of leading with care," Einterz says. "We always need to be asking ourselves if what we are doing is going to help build the health-care system in the developing country. Not to devalue research, but the mission of an academic health center has to be about changing the health system for the better."

Despite the program's focus on HIV/AIDS, the day-to-day leaders of AMPATH, are not infectious disease specialists but general internists. For Einterz, this lack of specialization by the partnership's leaders is a key to the program's success.

"It is not an accident that this [Indiana University commitment] blossomed in the Division of General Internal Medicine rather than a dean's office or another subspecialty department," he says. "It is also where Wishard's community clinics sprang from. It may be my romanticized view of internal medicine, but we tend to take a broader perspective on health and take more into consideration the needs of the community. We tend to be more astute than subspecialists in putting together systems of care. General internists bridge primary medical care and public health, which is important because in the U.S., there is a gap between public health and care that is unfortunate. To establish a partnership like we have done with Moi, you need to understand both domains."

AMPATH's leaders do not claim to have discovered the "silver bullet" that will solve all global health crises, but the significance of AMPATH's success may reach far beyond western Kenya. This type of academic health center partnership may be the most robust model for global health success yet discovered. Properly inspired to "lead with care," an academic health center partnership answers the call of development experts like Jeffrey Sachs for immediate mobilization to meet critical health needs, while simultaneously nurturing the kind of homegrown efforts that foreign aid critics like William Easterly cite as the key to sustainable success. Of AMPATH's more than nine hundred staff members in western Kenya, all but a handful, including nearly every physician and all the clinical officers, are Kenyan.

As the influx of PEPFAR support beginning in 2004 fueled AMPATH's growth, the program's success was beginning to get noticed. Jim Morris, former executive director of the UN World Food Program, which combines with AMPATH in feeding HIV-affected people, told an Indianapolis newspaper in 2006, "By training so many Kenyans and developing so much infrastructure, AMPATH is developing huge capacity for the country, and it is going to take huge capacity to handle this disease."

In early 2006, during his confirmation hearings to become the new administrator of the U.S. Agency for International Development (USAID), Randall Tobias told the U.S. Senate Foreign Relations Committee that his support for the AMPATH program was one of his most significant accomplishments in his three years as President Bush's AIDS czar. "Beyond attention to the current health care crisis, what Kenya has needed most—what Africa needs most—is help in growing its own health care capacity," Tobias said. "That's exactly what this program is doing, while at the same time delivering healing and hope. This is what transformational development is all about."

Commentators like Laurie Garrett understandably worry that aid programs focus too much on one or two diseases and don't integrate their efforts into the general public health systems. But Indiana–Moi's diverse services—including the nutrition programs, job and agricultural training, safe water efforts, care for orphans and vulnerable children, budding oncology and maternal and infant health programs—are all built on an infrastructure created in part by HIV-focused aid.

This is not always the case, as increased attention to African poverty and disease has inspired a variety of small-scale and short-term efforts by health-care workers from the United States and other developed countries. In her *Foreign Affairs* article, Garrett warned that these initiatives, while laudable, have limited value. Indiana–Moi leaders agree. "Lacking institutional backing and without connection to a long-term effort, these approaches can not substantially contribute to the building of developing countries' health care systems," they wrote in their *Academic Medicine* article. In contrast, AMPATH's clinical care sites, eighteen in all by the end of 2008, are located in government clinical settings and staffed by Kenyan government representatives. AMPATH staffers typically are employees of either the Kenyan Ministry of Health (through the Moi Teaching and Referral Hospital) or the Ministry of Education (through the Moi University School of Medicine).

Is it possible for AMPATH's partnership structure and holistic-care approach to serve as a model for global health and development efforts? Some AMPATH supporters readily acknowledge the program's success, but question whether the partnership's achievements can be easily replicated. PEPFAR's Buck Buckingham points to the lessons learned and the trust developed in Indiana–Moi's decade-long partnership before it launched widespread HIV/AIDS care, and the "dynamic" on-the-ground leadership of Mamlin and Kimaiyo. "I wish there was a pill we could give to provide those kinds of qualities to other partnerships," Buckingham says.

AMPATH's leaders acknowledge the advantages they enjoy as a result of the mature Indiana–Moi relationship, and are quick to credit Indiana University's Division of General Internal Medicine for using clinical care income to underwrite Indiana's first years of Kenya expenses. But they also insist that theirs is a model capable of replication if funding is available to support such academic medical center partnerships, and if enough time is allowed to build knowledge and trust between the partners. "If you have a university and a national referral hospital willing to work together in an African country, they can make a similar partnership with a U.S. university," Kimaiyo says. "The key is to have the hospital and the school talking to each other, and not involving the care program in too much bureaucracy."

"It is ridiculous to say that Indiana–Moi cannot be replicated, because no one has tried to replicate it," Einterz says. "What if we created endowed chairs at three medical schools and told them to replicate what IU and Moi have done? It would be hard without the long-term relationship that we enjoy, and there would need to be a start-up phase. But there are research partnerships all over the world. What is preventing us from doing similar partnerships based on care?"

As Einterz says, academic health center partnerships between the global north and global south do exist, but they have largely been limited to research. This frustrates Joe Mamlin. "One of the great shames of international medicine is that academic health center relationships have been project-to-project rather than taking advantage of the centers' power to build sustained systems of care," he says. In their *Academic Medicine* article, Mamlin and his colleagues issued an explicit challenge to African and U.S. academic health centers, along with private and government funders, to address "the shameful fact that millions are dying of treatable and preventable diseases in the developing world."

They wrote:

> For African academic medical centers, this means discovering the dormant power that resides in the tripartite mission of patient and community service, teaching, and research. For U.S. academic medical centers, it means risking far more than collaboration in fully-funded research and training ventures, and instead engaging in a committed and equitable relationship with their developing world counterparts.
>
> It was an accident of epidemiology that caused our Indiana–Moi partnership to be confronted by the greatest pandemic of our time, but it is no accident that an academic medical partnership has been able to respond to the crisis quickly, comprehensively, and effectively. We call upon other academic medical centers in North America and Africa, and the funders that support them, to discover their own potential for a similarly meaningful response.

AMPATH IN ACTION

ON THE DAYS WHEN DR. CAROLINE KOSGEI sees patients at one of the three AMPATH clinics in the Mt. Elgon area, she wakes before dawn, kisses her eighteen-month-old son Jonathan good-bye while he sleeps, and heads out the door. If Kosgei is fortunate, it is a two-hour drive northwest from Eldoret to Mt. Elgon. But in the rainy season, when the dirt roads turn to mud and collapsed bridges slow progress and force detours through the mountain villages, she can expect to spend at least three hours in the jeep. Kosgei has to pass through three police barricades en route to the Cheptais clinic, which is so close to the Ugandan border that her cell phone display changes to "Welcome to Uganda."

A graduate of Moi University School of Medicine and a native of Eldoret, Kosgei, who is twenty-eight years old, is the medical officer in charge of these remote clinics. She grew up in a Kenyan middle-class household; her father works as an accountant for Moi University and her mother teaches at the university's nursing school. But their relative prosperity has not kept AIDS from hitting the family hard. Kosgei's uncle died from AIDS in 2001 in Nakuru, before AMPATH's treatment program had begun to grow. Six months later, the uncle's wife died too. While Kosgei was a medical student making rounds on the wards of Moi Teaching and Referral Hospital, she came across a neighbor in one of the hospital beds. He died of AIDS a few weeks later.

"Before AMPATH, the wards were just horrible," she says. "There was no specific way to care for the HIV patients." After emotionally wrenching days in the hospital, Kosgei and her friend and fellow student Rose Koskei would talk into the night, trying to help each other deal with the frustration of working with patients whom they could not treat. Together, they questioned the point of becoming doctors at all if they were powerless to stop such immense suffering. Even their fellow student Daniel Ochieng fell ill, and they watched him waste away like all the others before him. Caroline and Rose cried over Ochieng, and awaited his inevitable death.

But, miraculously, Ochieng began to gain weight and strength. After seeing the effects of the antiretrovirals on her friend, Kosgei rediscovered her hunger to be a physician. A post-internship year at a hospital in Nairobi, where there was limited and uncoordinated HIV testing and care, inspired her to return to Eldoret and work for AMPATH. Finally, she would get the chance to treat patients for the illness that had killed so many in her community. Rose Koskei joined AMPATH as well, and became medical officer in charge of the equally remote Port Victoria clinic.

But even with miracle drugs on hand, providing medical care in the developing world can be an enormous challenge. Kosgei discovered that truth in Mt. Elgon, where a long-running land dispute between two clans, the agricultural Soy and the hunter-gatherer Ndorobo, has led to clashes that have cost hundreds of lives and displaced thousands of people. On a Friday morning in January 2007, Kosgei's efforts to care for HIV patients became caught up in the violent feud.

"When I arrived at the clinic that morning, at about 8 AM, there were already eighty patients waiting," she says. "Friday is market day for the village of Cheptais, and all kinds of tribes— Tesos, Elgon Masai, and Ugandans—go to market that day. About thirty minutes after I started seeing patients, I heard loud noises and ran out of the clinic to see what was going on. There were people running through the clinic yard, carrying *panga*s [machetes] and screaming that people were being killed.

"Soon, people began carrying dead bodies into the clinic. Some were beheaded and some of those heads had even been crushed after they had been severed. The conflict was moving toward the clinic, so police came into the building and told us that we all had to pack up and go.

"I started packing up my things, but then I noticed something. All of my patients were still sitting there—they hadn't left even with all that was going on. I called Dr. Mamlin on the cell phone and he agreed with the police—I should go. But I just couldn't. The patients needed their care and needed their medicine. I could not leave when all of my patients were willing to stay." Kosgei unpacked her medical bag, asked the police to do the best they could in guarding the clinic, and resumed seeing her patients.

The next week, Kosgei moved the clinic to the village of Chesikaki, a safer location next to a police post. But some of her patients were too weak to walk the additional kilometers to the new clinic, and too poor to pay for a ride. Other patients had to avoid normal roads as they walked to the clinic, instead hiding in bushes and forests en route in order to avoid being attacked. The clinic relocation was the latest in a series of burdens for many of Kosgei's patients, who not only endured HIV but had been forced to abandon their *shamba*s [farms] in disputed areas. "If you are found on one of these pieces of land, you are killed if you are a man and raped if you are a woman," Kosgei says.

After just a few weeks, Kosgei reopened the Cheptais clinic, having decided that the risk of continued clashes had to be accepted for the benefit of patients who would die because they could not get to another site. Her husband, an anesthesiologist at Moi Hospital, tells her she should stop going to the tumultuous region. "It is scary," she admits. "But sometimes you just have to do it. I know my patients so well, I feel like I'm almost related to them. Some just have to see the doctor and then they feel better. So someone has to go."

Like all of the AMPATH Kenyan physicians, Kosgei has less hazardous and more lucrative options. She has worked at the Providence Portland Medical Center in Oregon and is well aware that many medical professionals have left Africa for the better pay and more comfortable working conditions of U.S. or European medicine. "We definitely can make more money in the U.S., but we are needed to help here," she says. "AMPATH is a good place to work because you can see that you are making a difference. AMPATH is making a huge difference."

❀

AMPATH's holistic approach to HIV/AIDS care has earned the program attention and praise. But according to the program's leaders, they really had no choice but to broaden the scope of their services beyond HIV treatment. They had to begin conducting routine chest x-rays and treating for tuberculosis, since the co-infection rate of HIV and tuberculosis was so high. There was no alternative but to address the nutrition needs of hungry patients like Salina Rotich or the income needs of impoverished patients like Evelyne Njoki. "We are in the business of reconstituting lives, not just immune systems," Joe Mamlin says.

So Mamlin saw no option but to treat Musa's malnutrition. In 2006, Musa was brought into AMPATH's Mosoriot clinic by his brother. Their home was so remote that Musa had to be carried for an hour before they could reach a bicycle taxi, and then finally a *matatu*, public transportation van, which brought them to the clinic. By that time, Musa, who was severely wasted from AIDS, was too weak to speak and Mamlin could not get a blood pressure reading. "For Musa, food became more critical than even his TB and HIV meds," Mamlin says.

Musa began a long in-patient stay at a mud structure that AMPATH built next to the clinic, and a regimen of donated liquid food supplement helped him put on weight. Mamlin says it was one of the happiest days of his life when he escorted Musa back up the mountain to his home. Or, at least, Mamlin escorted Musa until the patient pulled away from his doctor. "I couldn't keep up with him," Mamlin says with a laugh.

Most AMPATH patients are not as severely wasted as Musa, but as many as 40 percent of patients in some rural clinics need emergency food assistance. On a sunny morning in the fall of 2007, several dozen of those hungry patients line up in a field behind the Moi Teaching and Referral Hospital, where Felix Kiprono sits at a battered wooden table under a canvas tent. Before the day is over, more than 150 AMPATH patients will present themselves at this food distribution site.

One of those patients is Mary Langat, whose weathered face contrasts with a bright orange head scarf and floral print dress. Langat hands Kiprono a green paper reading "nutrition prescription." After she was diagnosed HIV-positive a few days ago at the hospital's AMPATH clinic, a nutritionist interviewed Langat about her family's food needs. It turned out that she is the sole provider for six children, and there was almost no food in the house. She was enrolled in AMPATH's nutrition program, which will provide for her and her family's food needs for up to six months. If by that time her farm is not producing enough to support the family or she cannot find work, she will be a candidate for help through Imani Workshop job training, farm assistance, and maybe even eventually a micro-finance loan.

Kiprono finishes his short conversation with Langat. She stands up slowly and heads off to pick up her bags. "*Asante* [thank you]," she says wearily. Today, she will leave with a week's worth of maize, beans, corn-soy blend and vegetable oil from the UN World Food Program, and fermented milk, eggs, and vegetables raised on nearby AMPATH farms. As of late 2007, there were thirty thousand other people like Langat receiving short-term food assistance from AMPATH.

✾

By the natural light coming from the skylights far above the concrete floor of the Imani Workshop warehouse in Eldoret, Maxmilla Tarus and a dozen other women, some with children on their laps, sit at a long table. Their fingers covered in lacquer, they carefully roll small pieces of magazine strips into tight oblong shapes a half-inch long. They are transforming pages of *O Magazine* and *Conde Nast* into beads for necklaces that are sold to visitors in Kenya and in gift shops in the United States. Tarus has short hair, a broad forehead, and a ready if blushing smile. Maxmilla Tarus is usually quieter than her co-workers, who often laugh and sing as they work. But when telling her story, her voice becomes strong and clear.

Tarus, a member of the Kalenjin ethnic group, is the young-est daughter of a family of ten children whose father left shortly after her birth. She attended school until eighth grade, but then had to quit when her mother ran out of money to pay the fees. Soon after, Tarus married and gave birth to her first son, Denis. But Tarus's husband drank too much; one time he even fell into the cooking fire while drunk and burned himself badly. After he healed, Tarus decided to return to her mother's home, where she delivered her second son.

Tarus began having increasingly severe bouts of illness, and soon became so weak that she could not stand up, lift her head, or get out of bed for weeks at a time. After nearly a year of ever-declining health, Tarus was carried to the hospital for testing. When the nurse told her she was HIV-positive, one of Tarus's brothers and one sister got up to leave. "What can we do? She is going to die," they said.

But Tarus's eldest sister continued to carry Tarus every two weeks to the AMPATH clinic at Moi Teaching and Referral Hospi-tal. Slowly, Tarus began to improve. Then she learned the news that hit her harder than her own diagnosis ever could: eight year-old Denis was HIV-positive, too.

"That was the day I lost hope," she says. Tarus was suicidal, but realized she was still too weak even to kill herself. She worked to get stronger, with the goal of taking her two sons to a nearby bridge over the Sosiani River and jumping off to their deaths.

But Denis kept encouraging his mother to get out of bed and take walks with him, and Tarus began to realize that not only was the HIV-positive boy still strong and healthy, he was exception-ally bright. He didn't know it, but Denis was convincing Tarus that there might be hope for the future. "He saved both of our lives," she says.

Tarus was also helped by joining a support group at the AM-PATH clinic, one of dozens where HIV-positive people gather to share the struggle. Tarus looked forward to the sessions, and she felt energized by the mutual support in confronting the stigma and stress of living with the disease. Tarus began openly acknowl-edging her HIV status and even joined a group that visited local schools to raise awareness of the disease.

After every support group meeting, Tarus would pass by the AMPATH Family Preservation Initiative offices. Soon she asked to be referred there for job training. She was thrilled to realize that she was again strong and steady enough to put thread through a needle. She found a niche making beaded ribbons in the workshop, earning several dollars a day and supporting her family for the first time in years. By 2006, Imani Workshop had expanded to a new space and created a separate department for bead making. A proud Tarus was named the manager of the new department.

She still struggles with how she is going to tell Denis, now ten years old, that he is HIV-positive. The boy is already starting to ask why he has to take several pills a day, pointing out that his younger brother, who is HIV-negative, doesn't take pills. Even though she is not sure how to deliver the news to Denis, Tarus has a clear message to other HIV-positive adults. "Accept your status, and life can go on," she says. She tells American visitors that she has a message for them, too: "Help other people like me. There are many more like me, and they need help, too."

✻

In a rectangular room on the second floor of the AMPATH Centre of Excellence for HIV Care in Eldoret, Judy Rafira asks the twenty-two people sitting on white plastic chairs to stand up and gather in the center of the room. She places a laminated copy of the Serenity Prayer ("God grant us the serenity to accept the things we can not change . . .") on the linoleum floor in the middle of the circle and all hold hands and recite the prayer together. When they sit back down, she speaks up again. "My name is Judy, and I'm HIV-positive." With that, the meeting of an AMPATH support group has officially begun.

The sharing starts slowly, until Cynthia, who looks to be no more than twenty years old, confides that she is very worried. Her CD4 cell count had risen only to 150, below the 200 level considered healthy, despite several months of antiretroviral treatment. A man across from Cynthia reassures her, saying he had started treatment with a CD4 cell count of 50. A woman at the end shyly says she was diagnosed at her first clinic visit with HIV after showing a CD4 cell count of only 12. "Whew," said the man who had first spoken. "You should have been dead!"

The conversation shifts when a young man asks if it is safe to smoke cigarettes while on antiretrovirals. He says that smoking seems to relieve his stress, which leads several people to talk about how stress affects their health. The psychological strain of being HIV-positive, not to mention often poor, hungry, and unemployed, helps explain why there are more than twenty-three thousand AMPATH patients who regularly attend these support group sessions.

Studies of HIV-positive persons in Africa show that more than 50 percent suffer from significant mental illness connected with their disease, with the top diagnoses being depression, substance addiction, and post-traumatic stress disorder. AMPATH's support groups help take the edge off the suffering in a format that takes advantage of the Kenyan cultural tradition of often working out problems in group settings. Like Judy Rafira, all of the AMPATH-hired group facilitators are HIV-positive themselves. Indiana and Moi doctors hope to someday raise the funds to train and hire more psychological staff, who are especially needed when patients face particularly tough issues like rape, the death of a family member, or the suicide of a fellow HIV patient.

This session grows lively when Mary challenges Sofia over a critical issue for Kenyan women living with HIV. Both women had husbands who refused to get tested or wear a condom, even after their wives had tested positive. Mary left her husband and moved back in with her parents. Sofia decided to pursue what she called a "secondary virginity": refusing to have sex with her husband. "That is not right!" Mary says. "Sex is a natural thing, and it is wrong to be in a marital bed without sex." Both turn to the men in the room, demanding an explanation why having sex without a condom is so important to males. A few of the men look embarrassed by this confrontation, but one explains there is a significant loss of feeling with condoms, although he says he wears one now. The group agrees that the condom issue has affected many of their marriages, and ended several of them.

The session breaks up a full two hours later, when the room is needed for a counseling session for "discordant couples" (in which one spouse is HIV-positive and one HIV-negative). AMPATH has special group sessions for widows and widowers, children with HIV, couples, and "Happy Hour," a group for people who struggle with alcohol abuse.

"The alcohol abuse rate in Kenya, and in East Africa in general, is sky high," says Indiana University physician John Sidle. A 2003 survey of HIV-positive and HIV-negative patients showed that over half of them reported alcohol consumption levels that could be qualified as hazardous. "And alcohol's toxic interaction with HIV is clear on many levels," Sidle says. "Alcohol contributes to a decrease in good judgment about risk behaviors, it acts as an immune suppressant that can increase the chance of catching the virus and accelerate the virus's effects, and alcohol decreases adherence for those who are on treatment."

Sidle is the Indiana physician who had left Kenya in 2000 struggling with his own alcoholism and in despair over the untreated AIDS patients overwhelming Moi Teaching and Referral Hospital. Sidle had also been on the steps of the U.S. Embassy in Nairobi on August 7, 1998, when an al Qaeda–linked bombing claimed 213 lives. After his difficult tenure in Kenya, Sidle returned to Indiana, settled into work as an emergency room physician and pediatrician, and expected never to visit Kenya again.

But Sidle finally agreed to return to Kenya in 2003 for a short visit to help set up AMPATH's new research office. During that visit, he saw a Mosoriot patient named Lydia transformed from a near-death skin-and-bones AIDS victim to a happy and healthy young woman. Sidle realized that there was now hope in Kenya, and he signed on to become one of the directors of research for AMPATH. After returning to Kenya, Sidle and his Kenyan AMPATH colleague Claris Ojwang created Happy Hour to address the needs of AMPATH patients facing their own addiction issues.

"John became a real leader for us, and deserves a lot of the credit for the success of AMPATH," Einterz says. "He oozes humility and he couples that with compassion and loyalty, which has always led to strong relationships with our Kenyan colleagues." For his work treating patients in the AMPATH Burnt Forest clinic and initiating prevention and treatment outreach to the commercial sex workers and truck drivers who present the greatest risk to spread the disease, Sidle was named a "Health Care Hero" by the *Indianapolis Business Journal* in 2007.

❀

One Friday afternoon in December 2006, after Joe Mamlin finished seeing his last patient at the AMPATH clinic in Turbo, he was picked up by Benjamin Andama, co-director of AMPATH's Family Preservation Initiative. The two men drove into the countryside, their four-wheel-drive jeep climbing in and out of deep ruts and holes in remote roads that are more often traveled by cattle than by vehicles. Finally, they reached a small farm, where a man in his thirties hurried up to the car, smiled, and stuck out his hand toward Mamlin.

"November 6th, 2004!" he said. Mamlin looked at him in puzzlement until the man explained that he was Ronald Kegoli, and that it was on November 6th that he finally found the courage to come see Mamlin at the Turbo AMPATH clinic. By that time, Kegoli's wife had already died from AIDS and his own deteriorating health was making it difficult for him to farm his small plot of land and support his children.

"I had seen this grim scenario many times over—loss of spouse, loss of resources, loss of hope," Mamlin says. "Our drugs began to do their magic with Ronald, but he was living proof that drugs alone are not enough." Even after Kegoli had regained his strength, he struggled to feed his children from the meager $300 he earned from his annual maize harvest.

So Kegoli enrolled in an AMPATH farming cooperative called Amkatwende, which means "rise up, we go." With the help of seedlings and expertise from the cooperative, and Kegoli's own exertions for several hours each day on a Stairmaster-type irrigation pump he calls "the moneymaker," he is now a successful passion fruit farmer. Kegoli's half acre of vines, which should produce fruit continually for seven years, earn him more than ten times his previous farming income.

❀

Veronicah Kosgei, an AMPATH community health worker, leads visitors through an Eldoret slum, where plastic litter melts into red mud and goats pick at the contents of trash heaps. A small boy, naked from the waist down, stands in the middle of the road, urinating.

Kosgei stops at the door of one of the many ten-by-ten-foot shacks with tin roofs, mud walls, and no running water or electricity. *"Hodi!"* she calls, the traditional Kiswahili request to enter a house or room. *"Karibu"* comes the answer—you are welcome here. In the dark room, a young woman sits on the bare earth floor, holding a baby in front of a sack of grain stamped with "WFP"—World Food Program.

"This home is child-headed, both parents are dead," Veronicah tells the visitors. "The older brother takes care of his four younger siblings, but has not been able to find work. This is his wife, she is eighteen and also comes from a child-headed home. That is her baby."

The ravages of the AIDS pandemic on people of childbearing age has left Kenya with an estimated two million AIDS orphans. Kosgei makes about fifty of these home visits a week. She sees grandmothers caring for seven children because the children's parents have died, widows raising their six children and another half dozen orphaned nieces and nephews, child-headed households where fifteen-year-olds become the parents to their younger brothers and sisters. Many of these orphaned children are HIV-positive themselves. Kosgei and AMPATH provide food, blankets, school fees, uniforms, and other necessities to four thousand children enrolled in AMPATH's Orphans and Vulnerable Children program.

Kosgei was a health-care worker for the Catholic church before she joined AMPATH, and has taken in a homeless child to live along with her own three children. "I feel it is in my blood to take care of orphans and street children," she says. Kosgei knows from hard experience that she can't save every child she reaches out to, but she also knows that there is untapped potential in even the poorest child. One of the first orphans she helped is also one of her favorite success stories. "He is now studying medicine in Nairobi," she says proudly, "and provides for a wife and son of his own."

At the same time, Kosgei's colleague Margaret Acegwa is making similar home visits in the rural area around the village of Turbo. As she walks up to the open door of the mud-walled hut owned by David and Felicia Bwonde, Acegwa steps between two of the three graves in the front yard. The graves are fresh enough that the red dirt is still rounded with only a few weeds sprouting up. All three graves are surrounded by crude fences made of tree branches. In a disturbingly accurate microcosm of the Kenyan countryside, the Bwonde family is missing an entire generation. Their daughter Rose, their son Gelshom, and their daughter-in-law are all dead from AIDS and buried in the front yard, leaving ten grandchildren in the care of the Bwondes.

The two youngest children, Benedict and Sally, play on the floor of the hut below framed pictures of their parents, which share the wall space with a 1999 calendar featuring a picture of the Last Supper. Sally crawls up to her grandmother and into her lap, playing with a cardboard box that says "Epivir." Epivir is an antiretroviral drug—both children are HIV-positive. "We bring the children to the clinic in Turbo, but they are not getting better," David Bwonde says. "Sometimes they are OK; sometimes they fall down."

David Bwonde thanks Acegwa and her American AMPATH colleague, former Peace Corps volunteer Tomeka Peterson. AM-PATH helped with fertilizer and seed for Bwonde's recent maize crop, which yielded ten bags of corn that should last the family for several months. AMPATH has also brought a much-needed blanket for the children, and treats all of the Bwonde orphans who are HIV-positive. Two thousand orphans receive such assistance from AMPATH, and several thousand more receive food assistance alone.

But the family's situation is still precarious. Bwonde owes 15,000 Kenyan shillings in unpaid bills from his son's hospitalization before he died, and the hospital is holding Bwonde's government identification card and title to his land as collateral. With his rocky land mostly unsuitable for tilling and every spare shilling going to the children's clothing and school needs, Bwonde has no way to pay the bill, which comes to almost $255 in U.S. dollars. He shrugs his shoulders. "It is another problem that I have, but I do not hear angels from heaven coming yet."

❋

A young woman patient walks up to the open-air rural health center and answers some basic questions posed by AMPATH employee Rosebella Korir. Korir enters the information into a computer—which has a solar-powered generator backing up the sketchy electricity source—and prints out a small blue plastic card which contains the woman's name, village, and ID number. At the same time, about thirty feet away, an AMPATH clinical officer is filling out a form with more detailed health information on another HIV-positive patient. Down the road in Eldoret, a dozen AMPATH data-entry staffers sit in a small room on the top floor of the AMPATH Centre, typing into their computers similar medical observations recorded at other clinics.

This is the source of the AMPATH Medical Record System, which contains a massive 40 million observations for AMPATH's nearly seventy thousand patients. While the scenes of patient questioning and data entry are not as dramatic as seeing a wasted AIDS patient come back to life with medical care, the latter can not happen without the former.

"Some people see money or time spent on a medical records system as taking away from drugs and treatment, but that is a false dichotomy," says Dr. Bill Tierney of Indiana University, AMPATH's director for research. "Records are part of a health system—take away records from health care and it is like building a locomotive but making no track for it to run on.

"Especially for chronic diseases like HIV, you have to know the trajectory. What is the patient's CD4 count; what is her weight; what is her oxygen saturation; is she on first-line or second-line antiretroviral regimens? All of these factors come into play with every patient, and you can't know those details if they haven't been recorded somewhere and aren't available to pull up when the health-care provider needs it. If I am the doctor and I don't get that information, the patient gets lousy care."

Establishing a computerized medical record system in open-air rural clinics, which have no barriers to the elements or reliable electricity sources, posed obvious challenges. But Indiana–Moi's first-ever effort, with the Mosoriot rural health clinic, gained immediate results. The medical records revealed some previously hidden community health problems, including a village with far fewer vaccinations than others, a geographic concentration of rabies cases, and a cluster of sexually transmitted diseases. The solutions were simple: a nurse was sent to educate villagers and conduct vaccinations, the rabid dog was tracked down and shot, and the man at the center of the STD cluster was found and treated. But the simple solutions would not have been possible without computerized identification of the problems. A formal time-motion study showed that the computerized record led to a 23 percent reduction in patient and staff time spent waiting for care or on mundane tasks, allowing the Mosoriot clinic to double its patient and visit load without having to add new staff.

The electronic medical record system has benefits for research as well. With AMPATH forging new paths in HIV care, the electronic medical record allows the lessons to be shared through reliable and accessible data. "Research is learning something new, and the whole process of treating HIV in these settings is something new," Tierney says. "As new possibilities become available for treating unsafe water or protecting babies born of pregnant HIV-positive women, we have to evaluate these strategies to see if they will really work, especially in difficult developing world settings. Science is about dialogue, and one of the advantages of being an academic institution is that gathering knowledge to contribute to that dialogue is our raison d'être."

In 2004, the developers of the AMPATH record system teamed up with Harvard-based Partners in Health to expand their model into Open MRS, a free open-source electronic medical record which is now being used in Kenya, Rwanda, South Africa, Tanzania, Uganda. and Lesotho. To Tierney and the Moi–Indiana medical record team, the decision to make the software available for free to other African programs was a no-brainer. "We're not going to be making money from this," Tierney says. "I'm not in the software business, I'm in the making-health-care-better business."

✤

The current Moi Teaching and Referral Hospital maternity wards are grim places. Multiple women labor on spare benches just a few feet apart in the same small room, and then move to another cramped room where they deliver their babies, also in the company of other birthing mothers. But from these very rooms, the sounds of hope can be heard.

The sounds are the chiseling of concrete walls, the sanding of cabinets, and the roar of a cement mixer, all coming from the hundred men working on the new 38,000-square-foot Mother and Baby Hospital connected to the Moi facility. There is a critical need for improved maternal and infant care in western Kenya, where 13 women die of pregnancy-related causes for every 1,000 live births. There are visitors here from the United States and Canada, so Fabian Esamai, a pediatrician and dean of the Moi University School of Medicine, shows them the building in progress; he explains that it will be the site of up to 10,000 births each year and will include operating rooms for Cesarean deliveries and the first newborn intensive care unit in East Africa. As an extension of the Moi Teaching and Referral Hospital, the new facility will also provide for the training of medical students and staff, and enable clinical research for the benefit of mothers and babies in Africa.

The 40,000-square-foot AMPATH Centre, attached to the other end of the Moi Hospital, is the home base for HIV-focused training, research, and care throughout western Kenya. Similarly, the Mother and Baby Hospital will be home for a community-based program of maternal and child health. The Indiana and Moi leaders, joined by ob-gyn physicians from Duke University and the University of Toronto, plan to build upon the existing AMPATH partner relationships with traditional birth attendants, village elders, and community health providers throughout western Kenya.

This maternal and child health effort, along with ramped-

up cancer care—practically nonexistent for the poor of Kenya—
forms the core of a planned Indiana–Moi "lateral expansion" beyond HIV care. But without a PEPFAR equivalent to fund those
critical needs, private donors will have to support the effort, just
as they did—particularly Abbott Fund and Eli Lilly Foundation—
with the building of the AMPATH Centre and an operating theater
for Moi Hospital, and with the provision of care for rural AIDS
orphans. So, as Dean Esamai concludes his tour of the ambitious
new hospital, he gently reminds the visitors that the building has
yet to be equipped, and donations are still being sought.

❄

The landscape of the otherwise drab Nyao wards of the Moi
Teaching and Referral Hospital is dramatically interrupted by a
doorway framed with a rainbow-colored banner reading "Sally
Test Pediatric Center." Inside the door, three toddlers are eating
porridge together at a small red table next to shelves teeming
with children's books. A school-age girl is doing a math work-
sheet at one end of the room, while at the other end four adults
are making bottles and cuddling infants. Sarah Ellen Mamlin
hustles out of the room, headed to the grocery to refill the stock
of crackers and juice.

When Mamlin visited the pediatric ward at Moi Teaching and
Referral Hospital in 2000, she saw a barren area with nothing
but beds and concrete floors, paced by vacant-eyed children with
nothing to do. She began coming to these wards once a week,
bringing toys and games purchased mostly from departing missionary families.

"The kids would play with the toys and use the crayons and
scissors," she says. "These turned out to be fascinating foreign
objects both to the children and the parents. Often, the parents
would get down on the floor and spend hours coloring themselves."

But the setting of these sessions was not exactly up to western play-date standards. The only place Mamlin could gather the
kids together was in a hospital hallway where gurneys routinely
passed through carrying dead bodies. Then a gift from an India-

napolis philanthropist allowed Sarah Ellen Mamlin to drive a hole through a former hospital billing room, add on to the building, and create the Sally Test Pediatric Center, which now provides a place for pediatric patients' play and instruction. The center also hosts parent classes, provides a haven for abandoned babies, and served as the start-up location and inspiration for Eldoret's first-ever rape crisis center, which has served rape survivors from eleven months to one hundred years of age.

Joe Mamlin says that Sarah Ellen's work is valuable not just for the children and mothers she serves, but because it keeps both of them equally engaged in the struggle they share with their Kenyan colleagues. "This is a rugged environment in many ways, and you never know when a car accident will happen on these horrible roads—Sarah Ellen had a bad one a few years ago—or something else will pop up that wouldn't have been an issue if we had stayed back in the U.S. in retirement playing with our grandchildren," he says. "But sometimes in the course of a busy day we pass each other in the hospital parking lot or in the hallway, each of us moving as fast as we can to make this whole thing work, and we just wink at each other. That wink means 'no regrets.'"

MOVING UPSTREAM

IT IS AN EARLY SUMMER SATURDAY morning in 2007, and the rainy season has arrived in western Kenya. The people who begin filing into the expandable conference room of the AMPATH Centre have hopped the puddles in Eldoret and forded the sudden roadside streams on the way in from the villages. Sixty-five people, a dozen Americans sprinkled among the Kenyans, track brick-red mud across the white linoleum floor.

Dr. Sylvester Kimaiyo stands at the front of the room, looks out over the leadership of the AMPATH team, and smiles. "Today marks a great milestone for AMPATH," he announces. Kimaiyo turns on a PowerPoint program, and reviews the accomplishments of AMPATH to date.

One of the first slides shows the number of patients enrolled, featuring a graph with a sharply upturned arrow. Since Patient #1, Daniel Ochieng, began receiving antiretroviral medication in the fall of 2000, AMPATH has grown to the point where the program recently enrolled its 50,000th HIV-positive patient. Eighteen urban and rural clinical sites have been opened across western Kenya, where nearly two thousand new patients are added each month. Those patients are recovering at a remarkable and demonstrable rate; studies show AMPATH patients consistently gaining weight and increasing their CD4 cell counts well into the third year of follow-up.

By this time, Kimaiyo has fully assumed the reins of Kenyan leadership of AMPATH. When Joe Mamlin made presentations in the United States about AMPATH, he would show a PowerPoint photo of Kimaiyo, the manager of the program, immaculate in a green suit and tie, pushing an AMPATH vehicle that had been stalled in the mud of a rural road. Sometimes Mamlin would also tell a story he says epitomizes Kimaiyo's leadership style. Kimaiyo heard a rumor that a respected leader in one of the rural communities AMPATH serves was criticizing the program, leading some of the people in the area to decline AMPATH services. Kimaiyo could not confirm the rumor, so instead of confronting this person, he visited her and implored her to help in AMPATH outreach. Happy to have her importance in the community affirmed, the woman ended up traveling the countryside promoting HIV testing. "I'm so impressed by his problem solving, his patience, and his reluctance to condemn," Mamlin says of Kimaiyo. "You add that to how bright he is and how hard he works, it is a dynamite combination."

Kimaiyo finishes his presentation and yields the floor to Mamlin, who points out that only a few years ago it was widely believed that African HIV patients would not be able to comply with strict antiretroviral therapy. He then announces that less than 4 percent of AMPATH patients have had their initial prescription fail and that many of those failures were attributable to factors unrelated to patient compliance. This, Mamlin points out, is a tribute not only to the conscientious AMPATH patients but also to the clinical officers and outreach workers who fill this room.

Mamlin ticks off the program's chief accomplishments: 50,000-plus HIV patients, 30,000 people fed each week, nearly 170,000 people tested for HIV each year. Indiana–Moi's electronic medical records system, the first of its kind in sub-Saharan Africa, is thriving. Where AMPATH once offered HIV/AIDS screening and felt lucky if four or five people showed up, the community mobilization team now holds rallies and running races and tests nearly a thousand people in a day. Thousands of orphans are cared for, rape victims are sheltered, and abandoned babies are taken in.

The meeting room itself reflects success: This Saturday's gathering is being held in the AMPATH Centre of Excellence for HIV

Care, Kenya's first facility dedicated solely to HIV care, training, and research. This morning's crowd is dominated by Kenyans, as scholarships for Kenyan medical students and financial security for faculty members are stemming the dreaded medical "brain drain" from this corner of Africa. The group also includes medical school professors from Indiana and Brown universities. The University of Utah has sent physician-professors and students to Eldoret for years, and the University of Toronto and Duke University are adding ob-gyn specialties to the ASANTE (America/sub-Saharan Network for Training and Education in Medicine) Consortium, which includes Lehigh Valley Hospital and Health Network and Providence Portland Medical Center. In 2006, Indiana University–Purdue University at Indianapolis (IUPUI) established a formal relationship with Moi University to nurture academic partnerships in social sciences, engineering, informatics, and other disciplines.

AMPATH's accomplishments have not gone unnoticed. The program has attracted significant grant support from the United States Agency for International Development, the President's Emergency Plan for HIV/AIDS Relief (PEPFAR), the Centers for Disease Control and Prevention, the Maternal-to-Child-Transmission-Plus Initiative, and the Bill and Melinda Gates Foundation, as well as generous gifts from individuals and foundations in Canada and the United States. The program has been featured in the international mass print and electronic media, recognized with humanitarian awards, and has been nominated for a Nobel Peace Prize.

After quickly summarizing this good news, Mamlin clicks to a PowerPoint slide reading simply "Are we successful?" He pauses a moment to let the question sink in, and then clicks to another slide, which contains a stark "No."

"I think we are losing the battle," he says. Mamlin reminds the group of the grim global numbers most of them already know: Nearly 40 million people worldwide are living with HIV, and an estimated 2.8 million lose their lives to AIDS annually. In sub-Saharan Africa alone, it is estimated that nearly 3 million people were newly infected with HIV in 2007. Even where antiretroviral therapy is undoubtedly saving tens of thousands of lives, such as in AMPATH's catchment area, the disease still runs rampant. "It is unlikely that even 15 percent of the adults in our areas know their HIV status," Mamlin says. "We just opened our newest clinic in Khunyangu, and 70 percent of the married women already presented themselves as widows. That fact alone assures poverty, hunger, and endless numbers of orphans and vulnerable children." He shakes his head sadly, then gazes across the room.

"As fast as we are running," he says. "We cannot treat our way out of this crisis."

Of course, AMPATH has long since ceased to limit itself to HIV treatment. For many patients and their families, short-term food assistance is followed by enrollment in an economic sustainability program that includes employment and training in a tailoring and crafts workshop, agricultural extension services, or micro-finance support. AMPATH has launched care programs for orphans and vulnerable children and victims of domestic violence. The leaders in the academic medical center partnership have been able to call upon their colleagues in other disciplines to launch new efforts in maternal and child health care, along with tuberculosis, diabetes, and cancer treatment. AMPATH's lateral expansion from HIV/AIDS care eloquently addresses the concerns in the global health community that programs like PEPFAR and disease-specific funding do not provide a foundation for broader antipoverty and system-building efforts.

Yet the HIV/AIDS crisis retains its grim distinction as the most deadly force in western Kenya. So Mamlin clicks ahead to the next slide, marked "HCT."

Home-based counseling and testing (HCT) for HIV/AIDS is not a new idea, Mamlin explains. The Centers for Disease Control has recently concluded an ambitious house-to-house project in Uganda, testing well over two hundred thousand persons for HIV, with a high rate of acceptance of testing. "Going to people with the tests provides enormous opportunity for prevention and education that are largely lost by the time they get to the clinic," Mamlin explains. The AMPATH workers in this room know firsthand, and research in both the U.S. and Africa has confirmed, that knowledge of positive HIV status often leads to dramatic decreases in high-risk behavior.

The opportunity to prevent the spread of HIV by home-based intervention is most dramatically demonstrated, Mamlin says, by the high percentage of discordant couples (where one partner is HIV-positive, the other is HIV-negative) seen in the Uganda project. Of all HIV-affected couples tested at home in the program, 63 percent were discordant. The AMPATH nurses at the meeting murmur to themselves in apparent surprise, so Mamlin asks them the comparable percentages of discordant couples among those tested at AMPATH clinics. Only 20 percent of the HIV-affected couples at the clinics are discordant, they reply, even though AMPATH's own research shows that over 50 percent of the couples tested in the community are discordant.

"We are getting to them too late now," Mamlin says. "When we don't see them until one [member] of the couple seeks treatment at the emergency room or clinic, we are way too far downstream to prevent the disease from spreading."

The good news, Mamlin says, is that AMPATH is perfectly suited to move upstream and prevent the spread of the disease. A robust care system is the perfect platform upon which to build the most effective prevention program possible, he says. The availability of antiretroviral treatment and long-time relationships in the communities served provides credibility that will allow AMPATH teams to move through communities providing counseling and testing.

Mamlin quickly clicks through a series of slides outlining a pilot program in the Kosirai division of Nandi district, which is served by Mosoriot Rural Health Center, the site of AMPATH's first rural HIV clinic. AMPATH has been providing HIV care at Mosoriot for almost six years and has strong ties with all levels of the Kosirai community, dating back to 1990, when Bob Einterz spent part of Indiana University's first year in Kenya living and working at the Mosoriot clinic. Mamlin says the goal is to provide home-based counseling and testing to every household in Kosirai division, which has a total population of forty thousand people. AMPATH will try to reach all persons more than thirteen years of age and all children of mothers who are HIV-positive or deceased, since those children are at risk of having contracted HIV during birth. From the Kosirai community, Kimaiyo, Mamlin, and

Einterz intend to expand HCT to reach all two million persons living in AMPATH's western Kenya catchment area.

"You don't hear much about bold moves in HIV care in sub-Saharan Africa," Mamlin says. "It is hard enough to simply try to bring up fairly traditional HIV care systems capable of managing large populations of patients."

"But thanks to your hard work," Mamlin tells the assembled team, "we are ahead of other programs when it comes to providing treatment. So it falls upon AMPATH to risk the next move into uncharted waters. Imagine what we will learn if this is successful: We'll learn how to mobilize a large community for voluntary house-to-house HCT, we'll learn a community's true prevalence of HIV. Yearly retesting strategies will tell us what risk behaviors are causing the new infections."

"The big pay off," he says, "can be best described by the 'seven *Pre*s.'" Then Mamlin clicks on to another slide, and walks through each point:

1. *Pre*-patient. "With HCT, we can expect the majority of our new 'patients' to be healthy persons with HIV. This will open entirely new opportunities to avoid unnecessary sickness and death in children and young adults. The unit cost per HIV-infected person discovered through HCT should be a fraction of the cost of care for current AMPATH patients, who usually only come to us when they are already very ill."

2. *Pre*-concordance: "If the CDC experience in Uganda is mirrored in western Kenya, AMPATH can expect to become far more engaged in the care of families before both partners are infected. This may be one of this pandemic's most compelling opportunities for prevention."

3. *Pre*-widow: "At many AMPATH sites, over 50 percent of married women present as widows at the time of their initial visit. We see too often that a widowed spouse can struggle to feed and support themselves and their children, especially if they cannot cultivate their land or maintain their jobs as a result of losing their spouse to AIDS. HCT presents AMPATH with the wonderful opportunity to preserve food and income security for intact families with intact assets."

4. *Pre*-PMTCT: "We are always very excited about successful prevention of transmission of the virus from a HIV-positive mother to her child. But even more satisfying than aggressive PMTCT [Prevention of Mother-to-Child Transmission] is the opportunity to keep women HIV-negative during their reproductive years."

5. *Pre*-orphan: "Successful HCT is our best hope in knowing which parents are infected and keeping them alive. Very few children of HIV-infected parents will become orphans if the parents can be brought into care early."

6. *Pre*-tuberculosis: "We will conduct TB tests on all the people we test for HIV if they have had an unexplained cough for three weeks or more. We all know that TB is what is killing our patients—HIV is setting them up and TB is finishing them off."

7. *Pre*-vention: "The data from the first round of HCT, followed by periodic retesting, can define precisely what is causing the disease to spread in the community, which can pinpoint the most promising interventions for primary prevention. The supporting community networks we are putting in place to sustain HCT are perfectly positioned as agents of change at the village level."

Mamlin pauses, and looks around the room. The AMPATH workers are silent, every eye on the white-haired man with the clicker. "I only have one more slide," Mamlin says. Then he clicks to show a screen that reads, in big block letters, "BRING THE PANDEMIC TO ITS KNEES."

"Can you think of any other way—without a vaccine, without miracle drugs—to do this? HCT is our best chance. And knowing this team, you can probably do this better than I realize."

❀

A few months later, in front of the Mosoriot Rural Health Center, Neftali Chebii climbs into the back of a pickup truck which already holds four other persons. All are carrying green canvas bags, manufactured at Imani Workshops and labeled with large gold letters "HCT." The truck drops Chebii and an American colleague off by the side of the road, where they descend a steep path between fields of tea, bananas, and beans. A cow grazes on some untilled areas, and a strong breeze rustles the leaves of the avocado and blue gum trees. Chebii leads the way over a stream bridged by half-rotted planks that shift under his weight, then up the winding path, through one wooden fence, and under another barbed-wire one. He finally reaches a tin-roofed hut where a chicken pecks at the dirt yard and three boys sort out drying corn on a sheet on the ground. Jacob Kirui, a thin, balding man with a wispy beard, comes out of the hut to greet Chebii and his American colleague.

Kirui agrees to let Chebii speak to him about HIV, and brings out chairs for the visitors to sit in the yard and talk. In a conversational tone, Chebii goes over how HIV is transmitted and the importance of testing. The two Kenyan men have a joking exchange where they agree that condoms are a necessary evil. Then, like over 90 percent of the people AMPATH has reached so far in this home-based counseling and testing program, Kirui agrees to be tested for HIV. He is not concerned about the result, he says, even though his wife is in the hospital right now. "I trust my wife," Kirui says. "But I will have a big question if it is positive."

Chebii carefully explains the mechanics of the testing—two different tests will be used, and a third version available if the first two are in conflict. Chebii answers several of Kirui's questions in detail. He takes between thirty and forty-five minutes for each home visit, sometimes longer if the test is positive and more intense counseling is needed.

Chebii reaches into his green bag and pulls out the test kits to show to Kirui, then stretches white rubber gloves over his hands and wipes Kirui's fingertips with an alcohol pad. "*Uchunga kidogo*," he says softly in Kiswahili—you will feel a little pain. He pricks Kirui's finger, draws a thin straw half full of blood, and places a drop on each of two test strips.

As they wait the fifteen minutes for the tests to reveal their results, Chebii enters Kirui's name, age, and village into a PalmPilot, which he has attached to a portable GPS system to record the exact location of a *shamba* (farm) that has no address. Back at the Mosoriot clinic, the data will all be entered into AMPATH's electronic record system. As Chebii works and they await the results, Kirui seems to be growing agitated. He gets up to use the bathroom and comes back, worrying aloud how he will tell the children if the test comes back positive. "Sometimes you are married and all is good, but then you find out it is not really true. Sometimes you are away and you find out that your wife had sex with someone else."

Kirui's neighbor, Simon Chirchir, walks over to greet Chebii. Chebii tested Chirchir a few weeks earlier, and now Chirchir solemnly hands his green AMPATH card to Chebii's American colleague. It shows that Chirchir has tested positive, and his first appointment at the Mosoriot AMPATH clinic is scheduled for the following day. His wife had left him several months before, he explains, and he had no idea he was HIV-positive until he agreed to the home test.

Finally, it is time when the test results should be clear, and Kirui and Chebii bend over to look at the plastic strips where the drops of blood had been placed. Both tests show single red lines: negative.

Kirui smiles broadly. "*Sawa, sawa,*" he says—all is OK. Chebii gives him a card that indicates he tested negative and arranges a follow-up test for three months later. Kirui says in Kiswahili to Chebii, "I am very grateful for you bringing this service to the country. Most people do not have the ability to go to the village to get tested, so we thank you."

Then Kirui turns to the American and switches to English. "I am very happy. You have seen my body, and it is OK."

EPILOGUE

LESS THAN TWO MONTHS AFTER JACOB KIRUI was tested for HIV in the countryside of western Kenya, over nine million Kenyans went to the polls to elect the country's new president and members of Parliament. Held once every five years, presidential elections are high-stakes affairs in Kenya. With the power to appoint judges, a cabinet, and the election commission, along with de facto control over the country's budget, Kenya's president has a constitutionally provided stranglehold on important decisions in the country.

Every Kenyan presidential election since 1992 had seen outbreaks of partisan violence. Former president Daniel arap Moi was particularly notorious for hiring young thugs to attack and intimidate political opponents and their supporters. But the elections of 2007 seemed to be bucking that violent trend, despite the prospects of an extremely close race between incumbent president Mwai Kibaki and challenger Raila Odinga. On December 27, Kenyans came out to vote in record numbers, and international observers and Kenyans alike reported that there were no significant barriers presented for the millions who lined up to cast their ballots. On the morning of December 29, as the votes were still being counted, Joe Mamlin wrote home to his colleagues in Indiana. "I feel something wonderful is happening in Kenya. There was every reason to expect chaos with these elections, but all is quiet. One can sense a combination of pride and excitement as Kenyans begin to sense the real power of their vote."

But just a few hours later, Mamlin sent a very different message: "Hold on a bit! I just made the mistake of trying to go downtown in Eldoret and that turned out to be impossible. People are running everywhere. Traffic rules were suspended as everyone began driving away from town as fast as they could." As Mamlin finished typing, a Kenyan colleague rushed into the Indiana University compound, having passed on his way two people with their throats cut lying on the side of the road.

The chaos followed disturbing news from the capital in Nairobi. The Orange Democratic Movement party of challenger Odinga had won a majority of the seats in the parliamentary elections, and among the defeated were several of President Kibaki's cabinet members. The early presidential returns confirmed the pre-election polls' predictions that Odinga would become the first candidate in Kenyan history to unseat an incumbent president. But the Kibaki-appointed election commission was taking a suspiciously long time to tally the presidential votes, leading to rumors of ballot box stuffing. As news trickled in, the concerns seemed justified: one polling center would announce 25,000 more votes for Kibaki than the tally reported on election day, and an election official claimed he was forced to verify inflated Kibaki vote totals. International observers would eventually conclude that the counting process was rigged.

On December 30, election commission chair Samuel Kivuitu announced that Kibaki was the winner. Within the hour and behind closed doors, Kibaki was sworn in for his second term. Riots immediately broke out in Nairobi, especially in Odinga's parliamentary district in the desperate slum of Kibera. Young men roamed the streets, burning shops and attacking those who they perceived to be Kibaki supporters.

Most of those who were rampaging in Nairobi were from Odinga's Luo ethnic group, and the targets of their wrath were predominately from Kibaki's Kikuyu group. Kenya's 36 million people are divided among more than forty ethnic groups, each with its own language and cultural traditions, although people from dissimilar backgrounds are dispersed throughout the country, share the Kiswahili language, and often intermarry. Despite this integration and Kenya's history of relative peace and prosperity compared to other East African nations, the election dispute appeared to be pulling the lid off a simmering cauldron of ethnic resentment.

Kibaki's Kikuyu community comprises an estimated 22 percent of the country's population, making it Kenya's largest ethnic group. The Kikuyu are trailed closely in numbers by the Luhyas, the Luos, and the Kalenjins. Most of the population of the Eldoret area in Kenya's western highlands is Kalenjin. Ever since Kenya won its independence from Britain and Kenya's first president, Jomo Kenyatta, installed members of his Kikuyu clan in most positions of influence, Kikuyus have controlled a disproportionate percentage of Kenya's power and wealth. While most Kikuyus live in poverty, many have been very successful in operating small businesses. Other Kikuyus purchased fertile land in the Rift Valley from the departing British, a particularly sensitive issue since only 20 percent of Kenya's land is arable and other ethnic groups had once farmed the acres that the Kikuyus purchased from the colonialists.

There is a large gap between rich and poor in Kenya, whose income inequality is ranked the 29th worst in the world according to the 2007/2008 UN Human Development Index. Within Kenya, members of the Kikuyu group are often referred to as the prime beneficiaries of that wealth gap. But it is probably more accurate to attribute much of that uneven distribution to the country's postcolonial legacy of official corruption, where political power seems to inevitably lead to fabulous economic gains. For example, the families of former presidents Kenyatta and Moi (a Kalenjin) own vast tracts of Kenya's most fertile land. The country that Kenyatta helped found has almost half its population living in extreme poverty and an unemployment rate of more than 40 percent, but Kenyatta's family alone holds claim to more than five hundred thousand prime acres.

Ironically, given that Raila Odinga himself is a wealthy second-generation member of Kenya's political class, his candidacy was seen by many Kenyans as a crusade to rectify the uneven distribution of the country's resources. When an apparent election victory was snatched away by the Kikuyu-dominated ruling party, many of Kenya's unemployed and desperate youth responded with mob violence, particularly in areas where Kikuyus were in the minority and the history of land disputes fueled the anger. Many of the mob targets in and around Eldoret were Kikuyus occupying land that had been traditionally farmed by Kalenjins, many of whom had supported Odinga. Even though some of the supposed ethnic land boundaries were a legacy of artificial colonial divisions, many angry young men thought the time had come to drive the Kikuyus out of the land some Kalenjin felt was still their own.

After the hasty announcement of the election results and the immediate surge of violence, AMPATH staff and patients began streaming into the Indiana University compound in Eldoret, seeking refuge. One patient arrived after seeing her husband killed with a bow and arrow and her landlady die from *panga* (machete) cuts. Others came in when their neighbors burned their homes down. Ultimately, 130 people would crowd into the five houses rented by Indiana University.

On New Year's Day, a few kilometers from the Indiana compound, a mob of young Kalenjin men roamed the countryside, rousting Kikuyu families from their homes, burning their property, and often attacking the inhabitants. Dozens of men, women, and children ran from their homes to huddle in the sanctuary of the nearby Kenya Assemblies of God Pentecostal Church. A gang of young men followed them, poured gasoline on the building, and set it on fire. At least thirty people died in the flames.

Many of the survivors, and some of the dead, were taken to Moi Teaching and Referral Hospital, where the burn victims were laid next to others bleeding from machete cuts. Mamlin heard the news of the attack and rushed to the hospital. "This will go down as the worst day of my life," he would write later. "In the emergency room, I step over the dead to reach for those dying." A Kenyan surgeon began triaging patients as Mamlin led caravans to obtain extra IV fluids and suture sets. As one caravan made its way to the Eldoret airport to pick up Red Cross supplies and an extra trauma surgeon, the vehicles passed burning shops and hundreds of refugees walking the road. Crude roadblocks

had been set up so that the gangs could force all drivers and passengers to identify themselves. Those from the "wrong" ethnic
group were pulled from their cars, and many were killed.

As he stood on the tarmac of the airport, Mamlin could see
smoke rising from all directions. Back at the Indiana compound,
which was now overflowing with those who had fled the chaos,
the refugees wondered aloud if Kenya was about to become another Rwanda, where 937,000 were killed in the notorious 1994
genocide.

After the bloody New Year's Day, the violence slowed but did
not stop. Subsequent investigations by the United Nations and
the advocacy organization Human Rights Watch revealed that
the first spontaneous bursts of violence were followed by organized efforts by political and ethnic group leaders to clear rivals
from disputed territory. One Kalenjin elder told Human Rights
Watch, "[The elders] said that if there is any sign that Kibaki is
winning, then the war should break . . . They were coaching the
young people how to go on the war." Predictably, those attacks
led to reprisals in areas controlled by Kikuyus. A young Kikuyu
man who participated in revenge attacks on Luos also spoke to
Human Rights Watch. "It was arranged by people with money;
they bought the jobless like me," he said. "We need something
to eat each day."

Members of ethnic groups which were minorities in their
home regions began to flee the areas where many of them had
lived for generations. In Eldoret, that meant that thousands of Kikuyus piled onto buses and trucks heading under military guard
to the Central Province area north of Nairobi, where Kikuyus
formed a majority. Others retreated to crowded camps for those
who had been left homeless or were too frightened to stay in
their homes. These scenes were repeated throughout Kenya until
an estimated three hundred thousand people were categorized as
"internally displaced" and U.S. State Department official Jendayi
Frazer accused Kenyans of engaging in ethnic cleansing.

One of Mamlin's Kikuyu patients approached him in the hospital before she headed for the trucks leaving town. She had been
burned out of her home and had only the clothes on her back.
Mamlin gave her some money, a month's supply of antiretroviral

medications, and three breakfast bars that were in his pocket. One AMPATH nurse was Kalenjin but married to a Kikuyu. Her husband and son were evacuated, and she slept each night on the lawn of the Eldoret police station, along with dozens of others who feared nighttime attacks. Rumors circulated that Kikuyu gangs would soon return to Eldoret to seek their revenge, possibly by poisoning the city's water supply.

But even in the midst of fear and despair, there were signs of hope for Kenya's return to peace. The Kenyans who had fled to the Indiana University compound were of a variety of ethnic groups and political leanings, but the disputes outside had little impact on the atmosphere inside the new community. Within the "IU House" gates, Kikuyu, Kalenjin, Luo, and Luhya shared cooking duties, rotated laundry room access, and cared for each other's children.

Each night, they convened a worship service, singing hymns and praying for peace and reconciliation. "They all sang together, then they all began to pray at the same time," Joe Mamlin says. "It was not like any prayer I had ever heard before. Likely each person there was from a different denomination but each prayed aloud simultaneously.

"It had a beauty that defined prayer. Tears rolled down all cheeks as the prayer of many voices transitioned into beautiful music. Every ethnic group now at war prayed and cried together in the IU compound. At the same time, all of the children were in another room forming a living carpet as volunteers read to them or played with them."

"I know church when I 'feel' it down deep," Mamlin says. "This was church."

One night, just before 4 AM, a frantic phone call came to the Indiana compound from a small Bible college in Kapsabet, about an hour's drive from Eldoret. There were rumblings that violence against Kikuyus was planned for the next day, and the school had three Kikuyu students who desperately needed to escape the area. But they did not have a vehicle, and even if they had one, the way out was studded with the roadblocks set up by gangs for the explicit purpose of searching each car for Kikuyus.

AMPATH employee Javan Odinga volunteered to take a vehicle and head for Kapsabet, even though getting caught in the car with the Kikuyu students would likely mean gangs burning the car and killing him and his passengers. Because of the early hour, none of the roadblocks were manned. For most of the trip, Odinga was able to slowly move the jeep around the boulders, railroad ties, and logs left in the dark road.

Then he came across a huge log set up as a roadblock. Odinga could not drive around it, and no normal person could possibly have moved the log out of the way. But Odinga happened to be a heavyweight champion bodybuilder—a former Mr. Eldoret. He got out of the car, leaned his muscles into the weight of the log, and heaved it off the road.

Odinga arrived in Kapsabet and quickly put the three Kikuyu students into the car, ready to hide them under blankets if the car was forced to stop. They were able to make it to the Eldoret airport before dawn, from which the students flew to safety. Hours later, Kapsabet exploded into violence. Cars burned and several people were killed. It is quite likely that these three Kikuyu students owe their lives to Odinga, a Luhya, who risked his own life to save them.

Other Kenyans in the area were taking risks by sheltering Kikuyus in their homes, and the Mamlins ignored warnings of danger to themselves as a result of the Indiana compound becoming a sanctuary. Kikuyu AMPATH workers drove the dangerous roads to reach Kalenjin patients; Kalenjin staff braved the hostile environment of Kikuyu-dominated displaced persons camps to search for missing AMPATH patients. One AMPATH clinical officer, Patrick Bundotich, was helping care for some of the wounded when he recognized a young patient as the person who had threatened him and stolen his radio during an assault on Bundotich's home. Bundotich treated the young man's wounds anyway, never mentioning the incident.

Henry Mutieri, a Kikuyu AMPATH staffer, drove through the towns of Total Junction and Makutano looking for missing AMPATH patients, despite the fact the towns had been partially burned and Kikuyus were being attacked. AMPATH financial officer Christine Chuani, an unmarried woman whose last name reveals her Kikuyu heritage, found humor in the midst of the troubles. She refused to evacuate Eldoret, instead reporting for work at the AMPATH Centre and telling her colleagues, "I will not change my name until someone pays the right number of cows!"

AMPATH needed all of that determination. In the first week after the postelection violence erupted, less than 5 percent of the program's HIV-positive patients were able to make it to their clinical appointments. In the village of Burnt Forest, Kikuyu patients living in displaced persons camps were unable to leave to visit the nearby clinic. Kalenjin patients feared passing these same camps on their way to the clinic. With missed appointments possibly leading to interruptions in taking antiretroviral medication and a resulting risk of drug resistance, the consequences of empty clinics were life-and-death. Dozens of AMPATH staffers were themselves forced to flee to refugee sites far away from their work posts. *Matatus*, the vans that form the backbone of Kenya's transportation system, were not running. Skeleton crews staffed the clinics, and prisoners from Eldoret were enlisted to harvest the ripening vegetables on AMPATH farms.

On January 4, Sylvester Kimaiyo called together all of AMPATH's leadership team, some of whom were spending their nights on the grounds of the local camps for displaced persons. AMPATH quickly created a twenty-four-hour patient hotline and devised a publicity campaign to distribute newspaper, radio, and television notices telling patients where they could get their prescriptions refilled. Staff members fanned out to the countryside and the displaced persons camps to reconnect with missing patients. Fortunately, none of the AMPATH clinics had been harmed in the destruction, and even the clinics in the hardest-hit areas never closed. Slowly, patients began to return, and within ten days most clinics were seeing near-normal levels of patient visits. A fund created to support AMPATH patients and staff who were left homeless by the violence quickly attracted more than $100,000 in donations from program partners in Indiana and throughout the United States.

Meanwhile, former United Nations secretary-general Kofi Annan was brokering talks between Kenya's rival political parties. As the negotiations on possible power-sharing ebbed and flowed, the climate of outright violence began to be replaced by one of quiet tension. Reports circulated that rival gangs were arming themselves for another round of conflicts, and armored tanks rolled into Eldoret. If the Annan-led talks broke down, most Kenyans and diplomats feared, the violence would not only be renewed, it would be more efficient and brutal than before.

Finally, on February 28, Annan, with Odinga and Kibaki by his side, announced that a power-sharing agreement had been reached. Kenya would create a new post of prime minister, to be held by the parliamentary leader of the largest party in the National Assembly. Odinga presumably would be the first to take this post after Parliament made the necessary constitutional changes. The agreement also called for two deputy prime ministers to be appointed and a Truth, Justice, and Reconciliation Commission to be created to address both the postelection violence and more enduring Kenyan injustices.

The agreement was certainly no panacea. The prime minister's role was not clearly defined, and there was no indication of how displaced Kenyans could reclaim their homes and farms, assuming they were willing to risk returning to areas where their minority status had so recently made them targets. Many Kenyan and international observers feared that the power-sharing agreement did not address the wealth inequality and the corruption that had fueled the violence. "The elections were merely a trigger for the crisis, with the subsequent mayhem simply symptomatic of wider leadership failure," said John Githongo, who had cited death threats as his reason for leaving Kenya and his post as President Kibaki's anticorruption adviser in 2005 after revealing a scandal in which millions of dollars in government contracts had gone to a sham company. Speaking to the *East African* newspaper, Githongo minimized the importance of the Annan-brokered agreement. "Putting all the belligerents into one government only buys time," he said.

But the agreement did seem to guarantee some interval of peace, which for many was cause enough for celebration. "Prayers are answered, civil war is averted and Kenya is preparing to rise to heights never dreamed of in Africa," a jubilant Joe Mamlin wrote back to Indiana. "With our Kenyan colleagues, we will reach for the sick and the poor and the marginalized to do our part to make sure the Kenyan dream is shared by all."

When the power-sharing negotiations seemed to be reaching their make-or-break stage, Moi University religious studies professor Eunice Kamaara convened a meeting of the university's female staff and students to discuss the impact of the recent violence. "Women are affected through rape and the killing of their sons and husbands, and the recruitment of their children to militias," said Kamaara, a Kikuyu who had herself been forced to flee Eldoret for several weeks during the worst of the crisis. On the afternoon of February 28, Kamaara was leading the meeting of over a thousand women when she received a text message saying that a power-sharing agreement had been reached. As a student spoke to the group, Kamaara stepped aside to call a friend to confirm the news. "I am actually watching it on TV at home," the friend told her. "They are preparing for the signing." Before the student finished speaking, Kamaara received another text message: "Now they are signing . . . They have signed!"

When the student finished, Kamaara took back the microphone and announced the agreement. The hall erupted in ululations, screams, and applause before the women joined in a tearful prayer of thanksgiving. Kamaara took the microphone one last time and congratulated the group, noting that their celebration was not dampened in the slightest by the fact that none of those present knew the terms of the deal. "Kenyan women love peace so much that we did not need to know the details of the agreement," Kamaara said.

INDEX

FRAN QUIGLEY

is Director of Operations and Development for the IU–Kenya
Partnership at the Indiana University School of Medicine in Indianapolis. He is a lawyer and contributing columnist for the *Indianapolis Star* and other publications.

PAUL FARMER

is the Maude and Lillian Presley Professor of Social Medicine at
Harvard Medical School and a founding director of Partners In
Health. Farmer has written extensively about health, human
rights, and the role of social inequalities in the distribution and
outcome of infectious diseases. His work is the subject of Tracy
Kidder's book *Mountains Beyond Mountains*.